THE OVERWEIGHT
MIND

THE UNDENIABLE TRUTH BEHIND
WHY YOU'RE NOT LOSING WEIGHT

D0834401

JAY NIXON

ISBN-13: 978-1545040720

ISBN-10: 1545040729

To Lori with love and gratitude.
None of this would be possible without you.

My why, my passion, my purpose, my mission is simple.
I have a burning desire to help people live their best life.

"Gratitude opens the door to... the power,
the wisdom, the creativity of the universe.
You open the door through gratitude."

– Deepak Chopra

Contents

What Is the Overweight Mind?

Did you know over two-thirds of American adults are considered overweight? Our country is bloated. Our waistlines are bulging. Hell, even the name of the institute that provides the weight statistic (The National Institute of Diabetes and Digestive and Kidney Diseases) could use some trimming. We are living in excess.

How do you reverse the trend? How can you get back to a healthy lifestyle, one enabling you to live as your best self at a comfortable and healthy weight?

You could alter your eating habits. You could hit the gym more often. You could change your physical life in countless ways, but I'm willing to argue those won't be enough to overcome our overweight culture.

The journey to a healthy lifestyle must begin by attacking your **overweight mind**. If you think your diet and exercise regimens are standing between you and sustainable health, you only have part of the equation. While your journey to a healthy lifestyle may have been slowed by burgers, fries, and a lack of exercise, the mindset floating between your ears could have been equally detrimental. Thoughts like:

"I'm not good enough."

"I'm not an athlete."

"My family is overweight; it's in my genes."

"I like food too much."

"I don't deserve to be in shape."

"I don't like change."

"I have bad joints, so I can't exercise."

Whether explicit or subliminal, thoughts like these are more of an obstacle to a healthy body than any bag of food you could get from a drive-thru window. Your conscious mind overflows with thoughts, both positive and negative. The negative thoughts—those that will never serve you as you attempt to better yourself—will weigh you down. Your subconscious mind is programmed with countless habits and rituals that can either help or hurt you. While your subconscious mind is on cruise control, mindlessly allowing poor eating and exercise habits, the conscious mind is beating itself up. The tandem of a negative conscious mind and a subconscious mind steering you blindly into obesity can be a dangerous combination. It will never allow you to improve. That dangerous pair won't allow you to create the change you seek.

The aim of this book is to teach you how to lighten the load. If you're among the two-thirds of the population that is overweight, chances are your mind plays a larger role than you know. This book will teach you how to shift your mindset, raise your standards, and change your psychology to promote a healthy lifestyle. Each chapter will detail a portion of your overweight mind needing adjustment and present action steps designed to make those changes happen. I'm not here to give you information; I want to help you create the healthy lifestyle you desire.

You deserve a healthy body. You are worth it. It's time for you to prove it to yourself!

Chapter 1

....

80% Psychology, 20% Mechanics

"A healthy outside starts from the inside."
–Robert Urich

Eat fewer calories. Exercise five days a week. Eat less sugar. Eat more vegetables. Mix cardiovascular training with weight training. Balance your macronutrient intake.

Sound advice, but it's all mechanics. Each statement is valuable and should be implemented as you strive to achieve a healthy body, but relying solely on mechanical habits won't create lasting and permanent change in your lifestyle.

Mechanical changes to your lifestyle like the ones listed above are important, but not nearly as important as any psychological or mental shifts you make. In fact, when it comes to the breakdown of a permanent, happy, and healthy lifestyle, I'd argue mechanics make up about 20% of it. That's right, 80% of your health and wellness depends on your psychology or mindset.

I can sense some of you may still be on the fence about this ratio favoring your mental state, so let's consider some familiar examples to paint the picture. Have you ever seen *The Biggest Loser*? Even if you haven't watched a season from beginning to end, I'm sure you've at least read an article about some of the amazing transformations. Or maybe you've tuned in for a season finale where triple-digit weight losses are the norm. Watching these contestants work their asses off and lose so much weight is inspiring. The incredible transformations are the reason the show has stayed on the air for so long.

We'd all love to think these contestants step off the stage after the final show and go on to live happy and healthy lives with their friends and families. Unfortunately, that's not the case for some of the most successful contestants. Ali Vincent, the first woman to win *The Biggest Loser*, sat down with Oprah after her big win and discussed her huge weight loss. On the show, Ali had lost 112 pounds. What she told Oprah was that when she got home from the *Biggest Loser* ranch, she didn't know what to do with herself. All of the structure, exercise regimens, and changes in diet were no longer present in her daily life. She didn't have a coach screaming in her ear to keep pushing it on the treadmill. Essentially, the mechanics of her weight-loss journey broke down.

So, what happened? Her meal plans became less strict, she didn't exercise as much, and she had the liberty to go out and have drinks with friends whenever she pleased. She ended up gaining nearly all of the weight back.

Ali is not alone. She is only one example of a long list of *Biggest Loser* contestants who had a tough time keeping the weight off. The National Institute of Diabetes and Digestive and Kidney Diseases followed season-eight contestants and found thirteen of fourteen contestants gained weight back after the bright lights of TV had dimmed. This study also disclosed that the contestants endured a significant slowing of their metabolisms during their rapid transfor-mations, making it even harder for their bodies to keep up with the demand to burn calories. Their slower metabolisms (coupled with a weight-loss plan far too focused on extreme diet and exercise) created a recipe that left the contestants closer to where they started than where they finished.

We don't have to look far for more health transformations skewing the focus towards mechanics than psychology and mindset. Consider people who opt for bariatric surgery. Bariatric surgery shrinks your stomach (either by using a gastric band to minimize it or by removing a part of it). Individuals undergoing the procedure are likely obese and have the best intentions. They want to live healthier. They don't want to die young. They want to shed the emotional baggage accompanying their excessive weight.

Some patients find success and report weight loss over the long term. Unfortunately, many patients gain the weight back over time. In fact, in a study done by the American Medical Association in 2015, nearly half of the bariatric surgery patients researched reported significant weight gain within five years of their surgery. Why? Mechanics. Reducing the size of the stomach is about as mechanical as you can get in terms of weight loss. *You literally wake up with a smaller stomach.* Yes, bariatric surgery is paired with counseling, but the counseling isn't geared towards understanding and shifting a patient's psychology. It's aimed at advising him/her about proper food choice, how much food to eat, and what exercise regimen to follow. Sound familiar? More mechanics.

Don't get me wrong. Changing the food you eat and the way you exercise is *essential* to achieving a healthy body and lifestyle. But what deserves greater focus and energy for a lasting foundation of health is your mindset. You can't lose 10, 20, 30 pounds (and keep it off) until you first focus on losing your limiting beliefs, negative thoughts, and emotional baggage.

Think about it. The same person who created the mess you're in—you—is trying to get you out. The same psychological you, anyway. In order to find some permanence in your weight-loss results, you need to change as a person. You need to change your mindset. Maybe you ate so much because you were stressed. Maybe you drank too much because you were sad. Maybe you didn't exercise because you convinced yourself you're not an athlete. The reasons holding us back and perpetuating bad habits are numerous. If you just change the mechanics of your behavior by eating less or exercising more, you still haven't addressed the underlying psychology that got you out of shape in the first place.

In truth, no matter who you are, the process and mechanics of your health will break down. Even the most elite athletes and top performers have off days. Maybe it's a birthday party or Thanksgiving dinner or a night out with friends. There is going to come a time when they eat too much and exercise too little. No one is perfect. The difference between these top performers and the average human being, though, is that their mindset and psychology picks them up when they fall. They'll wake up the next day and get right back to work without blinking an eye.

They won't spend time telling themselves how terrible they are or how they shouldn't have had so much food. For them, those moments of indulgence are the exception, not the rule. They feel deserving of a good body, they *are* willing to put in the work, and they *are* living a happy and healthy lifestyle. Eating a handful of Christmas cookies, skipping a workout, and drinking one too many glasses of wine are the exceptions. The exceptions will happen, but when they do, elite athletes and top performers have a rulebook—a proper psychology—to get them right back on track.

Your psychology and mindset are crucial for lasting health and wellness. Setbacks happen to *everyone*. No one gets a free pass. By taking the time to focus on your mental well-being, you will be able to bounce right back when you stumble. Instead of making "the donut in the morning" the rule, it will become the exception. You won't let one mistake build momentum into another. A proper mindset will stop the bad habit in its tracks and won't allow it to persist.

"Great, Jay. I get it. My psychology is important! But how do I work on it? How do I make it more positive? Where do I begin?"

In the words of Simon Sinek, *Start With Why*. Sinek wrote an entire book detailing how important it is to find your "why," and I couldn't agree with him more.

"What's a 'why'? What does that even mean?"

Well, *why* are you doing this? *Why* do you want to be fitter? *Why* do you want to change your lifestyle? *Why* is it important for you to lose weight? *Why* do you want to eat better?

You need to find out *why* you want things so badly. The deeper and more powerful "why" you have, the stronger and more formidable your mindset will be. I urge you to dig deep on this subject—don't be willing to hover over the surface. Let me show you what I mean:

Why do you want to get in better shape?

"I hate being overweight."

Why do you hate being overweight?

"I don't fit into any of my clothes."

Why does not fitting into your old clothes bother you?

"I used to feel good in those clothes. I fell in love with my spouse wearing those clothes."

Why do the clothes have such a strong connection to your spouse?

"I feel there's a 'disconnect' with my partner since I've let myself go. I want to get back in shape to feel better about myself, but also to rekindle the fire we once had. I want to get *us* back."

What's going to help create the mindset you need for a healthier lifestyle—the fact that you hate being overweight *or* your desire to breathe life into your marriage? I would bet big money it's the latter. With a larger purpose driving you towards a healthy body, you will be less tempted to grab a cookie, skip a workout, or eat a whole pizza by yourself. Those things will become the exceptions. The new rule will be working your butt off to save your marriage.

> *"The real voyage of discovery consists not in seeking new landscapes, but in seeing with new eyes."*
>
> –Marcel Proust

It doesn't have to be marriage that fuels you. It could be anything significant to you. Don't be discouraged if you feel your "why" isn't big enough. You'll find the more you commit to the process, the deeper your "why" will become. You'll find greater purpose for the things you're doing, the healthy habits you're creating, and the hard work you put in along the way. What will begin as something small like, "I want to lose 20 pounds" will eventually blossom into, "I want to lose weight so I can keep up with my grandchildren. I want to run around with them, play with them, and watch them grow up." What's important is finding something—ANYTHING—significant enough to get you started. Trust me, you will find deeper meaning and a stronger "why" as you build momentum.

I hope it's clear your psychology and mindset are going to play a bigger role than you think in your weight-loss journey. It's a massive but often ignored part of any healthy lifestyle/weight-loss program. In the next few chapters, we will dive deep into what parts of the mindset need adjusting and what steps to take to effect change. Since it makes up 80% of your success, you better believe we're going to examine everything floating between your ears so you can improve your life, your health, and your happiness.

Testimonials from the Thrive Tribe

From my clients at the Thrive Fitness Studio in Palm Desert, California, to the clients I train and advise online, I've met and helped thousands of people achieve their best selves through fitness and nutrition. I call this group of wonderful people my Thrive Tribe. At the end of each chapter, I'm going to pass the mic to a client or two whose experiences exemplify the essence of the chapter.

Meet Heather S.:

"I remember seeing women at my children's school who had gone through pretty amazing transformations. Though weight loss was part of it, I was more intrigued by the glow, a confidence in their step, and an enthusiasm

and energy that had been eluding me for some time. I asked them what they were doing, and kept hearing about Jay Nixon.

I had lost control over the creeping scale and had been feeling unhealthy for a long time. I had been to doctors, read the latest diet books, ordered the trendy cleanses, and half-heartedly "tried everything."

Jay's plan has food recommendations and recipes that made it possible to eat well without depriving myself. Though this was a huge step in my improved health, the coaching and mindset shift around food, fitness, and life have been the key for me. I had forgotten that I mattered, and Jay got me back in touch with my WHY. I now realize my being unhealthy and weak in mind, spirit, or body does not serve those I love. The confidence I've gained from this program gave me courage to make long overdue changes in my personal life for the better. I am grateful to be part of what Jay has created, and know I will be forever fit."

Journaling the Journey

One way I've found to lighten the load of the overweight mind is to write down some of the thoughts swirling around in my head. I journal every day and I ask the same of my clients. Journaling allows us to see our thoughts for what they are and to be intentional about reframing the negative ones. Each chapter will show a personal journal entry that follows the theme we covered. There will be space provided for you to do some writing as well.

Jay's Journal

Today I am mindful of all my words, thoughts, and actions. I am present in my decisions, and all of my choices will move me closer to my goal of being my best self. Today I am grateful for the opportunity to be my best self. Planning all my meals today has helped me to stay on program and focused on my progress. Being mindful of what I put in my body helps me understand why I feel the way I do. Healthy food = feeling great both physically and mentally.

Your Journal

_____

_____

_____

_____

_____

_____

Actions to Overcome the Overweight Mind

You know what I hate? When someone reads a book, nods along at the sound advice, then never does anything with it. I've been guilty of it myself in the past. But I wrote this book to inspire people to take action. Changing your mindset is one thing, but your life won't change until you put that new mindset in motion. At the end of each chapter, I'm going to provide action steps to move your life forward. Here's the format you can expect from each and every chapter:

POWER Action: This is a non-negotiable, physical, mental, or lifestyle action you need to implement in your life immediately. It will create positive change in your life in some incredible ways when you put it in motion.

SUPER Action(s): Each POWER action will be followed by one or two SUPER actions. Once you've implemented and put the POWER action to work, come back to these SUPER actions to supplement your success!

Here's your first round of life-changing action steps. Put them to work and I promise that you'll create amazing momentum towards your ultimate goal.

POWER Action Step: We spent a lot of time in this chapter talking about your "why." You know, *why* do you want to lose weight? *Why* do you want to change your life? You get the idea by now. Grab a piece of paper or a notebook and spend 20 minutes journaling your thoughts about your "why." Try to break it down to its most meaningful level. If you're stopping at "I want to lose 10 pounds," you're not digging deep enough. Find the purpose driving you to success.

My Why:

_____

_____

_____

SUPER Action Step: Create a "word of the year" for yourself. Think of one singular word representing what you want to accomplish in the next 365 days. Use it to remind yourself of your goals—your destination. My word for this year is *connection*. My goal in writing this book is a desire to *connect* with as many people as I can and to help them make positive changes in their lives. Find a word to use as your driving force. Write it down where you can see it. Reflect on it every day and make sure your pursuit of that word is continuous.

Word of the Year

_____

Chapter 2

We Are Our Habits

We are what we repeatedly do. Excellence, then, is not an act, but a habit.

–Aristotle

Say it with me: We Are Our Habits. One more time: We Are Our Habits. Think about what you do every morning when you wake up. How much thought goes into every move you make as you wander around with your eyes half open? Do you have to make a critical decision about brushing your teeth? Do you have to weigh the pros and cons of taking a shower before you decide it's a good idea? Do you have to read the instruction manual on the coffee maker to make sure you're brewing correctly?

Doubtful, right? So much of what you do every single day is a habit, ritual, or pattern built into your brain over time. One last example to prove it to you. You get in your car to go to work, the grocery store, or someplace you've been hundreds of times. How hard do you have to think about each turn, exit, or road to take? Not at all. Sometimes you arrive at your destination and realize you'd been so busy sipping your coffee, talking on the phone, and fiddling with the radio that your brain didn't do much of anything to help you get there. It's as if you could've driven with your eyes closed. You were on complete autopilot.

The car ride is a metaphor for your life and your goals. There's a destination, a place you want to go, but in between your starting point and the finish line is a laundry list of habits you employ to get there.

Problem: your habits kind of suck. Don't take it personally; nobody's immune from a few persisting bad habits. If you're trying to create permanent healthy changes in your life, though, you're going to have to overhaul the patterns currently guiding you to an unhealthy dead end.

The seemingly innocent but unhealthy rituals you subconsciously perform every day eventually add up to an unhealthy body staring back at you in the mirror. If you go to the movies, you probably cozy up with a big bucket of popcorn and a large sugary soda. You're not alone. How about Thanksgiving or Christmas? Hell, how about the entire month between the two holidays? The holiday season presents infinite amounts of cake, cookies, and pie. But hey, it's the holidays. Everyone else is having an extra slice of grandma's pie, why shouldn't you? Because you don't have to. It's a habit you can change, and with my help, I hope you will.

There are plenty of habits that put you on autopilot throughout your average day, habits that, if changed, can dramatically improve the quality of your health. Here's the tricky part: you can't just "unsubscribe" from a habit as if it were an annoying email campaign from Bed Bath & Beyond. No matter how great your willpower, you can't simply eliminate a habit or an action from your subconscious mind (the guy or gal who's really running the show) without replacing that ingrained pattern with something else.

In his incredible book *The Power of Habit*, Charles Duhigg goes into great detail on how to alter or replace a habit. Essentially, for every habit you have, good or bad, there is a three-part "habit loop." First, the cue for your habit—the event or circumstance triggering the pattern. Next, the routine—the acts you perform. Finally, the reward—the way you feel or what you get out of performing said act.

The key to changing your habits, says Duhigg, is identifying and stabilizing the cue and the reward, while swapping the routine or the action for something more positive. Let's take a look at two potential habits and how we could change them for the better.

Your Morning Treat

Wake up! It's time for breakfast. Your alarm goes off, you start running around the house to get ready for work, pour your coffee, and grab a donut before you take off. It's quick, it's easy, and it's just one donut, right? Wrong. It's a bad habit, and it can be converted into something healthier with a little work.

First, what is the cue for your daily donut? Is it the morning rush around the house? Is it the fact you woke up hungry and need a quick fix? Is it the smell of (not so) fresh donuts emanating from the kitchen? Whatever the case may be, do some internal research and try to identify the actual trigger for your behavior. It may take some trial and error, but be honest and figure out what causes your action.

Next, identify the reward your get from eating the donut. Satisfaction of your hunger? A sweet treat? The only person capable of telling you *why* you're eating the donut every day is you. Don't judge the reward, just figure it out so you can use it as feedback for changing the habit.

Finally, identify the routine or the action and try to swap it with something that will serve you better. This should be the easiest part to identify because the action is concrete.

Let's review:

Cue: Morning rush

Routine: Eating a donut

Reward: Satisfying hunger quickly

The objective is to swap out the routine while keeping the cue and the reward in place. The routine is the easiest piece of the puzzle to replace, while the other parts—the cue and the reward—can prove more difficult to alter.

You are in a rush in the morning. You need something quick. What quick and satisfying item can you substitute that will both reward and satisfy you?

I tell every client the same thing: swap your morning donut (or bagel, or bowl of cereal) for a morning protein shake. Thirty grams of high-quality protein will not only set a solid foundation for your nutrition for the rest of the day, but it will also provide a seamless replacement in your habit loop. A protein shake is easy to prepare and quick to consume. Whether you shake it up the morning of or blend it the night before, the quick and easy preparation pairs well with the given cue. It will also satisfy your morning hunger, which gives you the same reward as the donut. By swapping your sugary morning treat for a filling and nutritious protein shake, you can alter an early morning habit while creating positive momentum to start your day.

Ice Cream Escape

You had a bad day at work, you fought with your spouse, or your children are driving you nuts. What do you do? You head to the freezer and reach for a pint of ice cream. It's a subconscious reaction to stress or sadness, but in order to start living a healthy lifestyle, it's important to take control of the habit.

What's your cue? Stress, a very common trigger. Your reward? Ice cream tastes good, it calms you, and it makes you feel happy. Also, by making the choice to eat the ice cream, you feel like you have control. Since it seems you chose Rocky Road happiness, you find added pleasure.

Again, here's the hypothetical loop:

Cue: Stress of some sort

Routine: Eating a bowl (or a pint) of ice cream

Reward: A brief state of controlled calm and happiness

Now that you've identified the phases of the cycle, you need to swap the routine for something healthy. How can you react to stress in a way designed to result in controlled calm and happiness?

Exercise. Go for a walk or a run to melt the stress. When you exercise, your body releases chemicals called endorphins. Endorphins react with your brain to reduce the sensation of emotional or physical pain. Isn't science awesome? Making the decision to lace up your shoes and go for a run represents as much of a controlled choice as reaching for that pint of ice cream.

To facilitate your transition from "eater" to "exerciser," put your sneakers in view of where you keep your frozen treats. You raise the level of accountability because every time you are tempted to react to stress by reaching for the Ben and Jerry's, you will see your shoes, reminding you of the newly selected action.

Every single day our subconscious mind leads us into actions like the early morning donut or the stress-induced ice cream coma. Raised awareness will lead us towards altering those patterns. Habits are powerful, but with great power comes great responsibility. You can either let your habits cumulatively destroy your health, or you can create positive habits, allowing you to live a healthy and happy life.

Over the course of the next week, take inventory of the habits and rituals you perform throughout the day. If there is a persisting negative habit you'd like to change, figure out what triggers the action. What is happening prior to the "donut" or the "ice cream"? How do you feel after you indulge? Keep a journal of it all and find routines you can insert that will serve you better.

People do not decide their futures; they decide their habits,
and their habits decide their futures.

–F.M. Alexander

As much as changing bad habits is critical, introducing new habits can be life altering as well. The power of breathing new life into your day through the introduction of an empowering habit can be amazing. My Thrive Tribe and I have introduced a life-changing morning ritual.

We call it the **Thrive Three**. Every morning we take some time to do the following:

» Write down three things for which you are grateful.

» Decide on three positive actions you will take during the day.

» Give three hugs, three high fives, or three messages of encouragement to a friend or stranger. Any combination will do.

Three simple things every single morning will start your day in an incredible way. Let's break down why, starting with gratitude.

Reflecting on what you are grateful for starts your day with a reminder your life's worth living to its highest potential. You're taking note of the good in your life, which subconsciously pulls you towards more good things throughout your day.

You can't be fearful and grateful at the same time.

–Tony Robbins

You can't be fearful, negative, or pessimistic when you reflect with gratitude. It is the antidote to your "I can't do this" mindset. Gratitude sets an amazing tone for the day.

Next, we decide on three positive actions that will shape our day. Reflection is great, but taking action is equally important. By choosing three actions in the morning, we are giving ourselves expectations for what we want to accomplish. Once we have decided on three actions, we know exactly what we need to get done, and we have a rubric to refer to if our day wanders off track. We can constantly refer back to the three daily actions to keep ourselves in line with our goals.

Finally, we want to spread love, encouragement, and positivity like crazy. Transferring positive vibes from yourself to another human via a hug or a high five not only makes you feel great, but it will also perk up the person with whom you interact as well. If all of us reach out to one another with, "Have an amazing day," or "I know you had an off day yesterday; today's a fresh start," we create ripple effects of positivity and reach numerous people.

Here's the best part: the Thrive Three only takes about ten minutes. It's not a two-hour study of your life or a deep reflection of your past. It's not creating a list of ten things you must do before you go to bed. It's not about reaching every human being on the planet. It's just taking about ten minutes to be present in three meaningful tasks to set a purposeful foundation for your day.

Notice—these three tasks have nothing to do with the physical body. People pay me to help them lose weight and to improve their health, but I require them to do this to start every day. Why? Because, as this book will continue to show you, the health of the body follows the health of the mind. The Thrive Three is a way of getting your mind right to begin each day. If you start well, I can help you tackle the mechanics of health and fitness in a more powerful way.

Let's refer back to the example of subconscious habits that I mentioned earlier—the car rides to work, the grocery store, or the mall essentially completed on autopilot. Your car pulls out into the road, some time passes, and you eventually reach your destination. What happened between the point of ignition and when you parked is a foggy memory, but you still got there safely.

It wasn't always that way, though, was it? At one time, you had to focus on each tap of the brake, each turn, and each signal. Your early days of driving required a lot of conscious effort. Your early intentional focus created good habits, eliminated bad ones, and honed your skills with each car ride. Over time, the habits you created led to smooth, steady, nearly unconscious rides from here to there. But your early days were essential to your success and safety as a driver.

In terms of living a healthy lifestyle, think from the perspective of a young, teenage driver behind the wheel. You need focus. You need conscious effort. Like a young driver learning the rules of the road, you need to be aware of the circumstances around you and choose how to deal with them proactively. Stay focused on your goal—remain mindful of each and every nutrition decision, and finally, be aware of temptations and unhealthy actions that can lead you into trouble.

Focus and you will eventually harness the power of habitual action for good instead of letting it wreak havoc on your health and wellness. I say "eventually" because habits aren't built overnight. It didn't take one or two trips around the block for you to master the skills of driving a car; it took hundreds, maybe even thousands.

Creating or changing your mental and mechanical habits will be no different. It will take time and conscious effort to create permanence in your healthy habits, so be patient. You've probably heard it takes 21 days to form a habit. The truth is, it could be less, or it could be more. In a 2009 study performed at the University College of London, students were asked to create and pursue exercise and diet goals for an open-ended amount of time. While these students worked towards their goals, researchers documented at which point habits formed throughout each individual journey. On the low end, it took one student only 18 days to create habitual change. That's amazing! You could stick anything out for 18 days, right?

The researchers also discovered it took some participants more than 200 days to create a formidable habit. That's right; some students took the better part of a month, while others took the better part of a *year* to form the healthy habits they sought. On average, the students saw habit change occur around the 66th day of the study—the sweet spot of habit change or creation.

I don't share these statistics to scare you. I merely want to give you the facts. By now, I think you realize that I'm not a "quick fix" kind of guy. Shortcuts and life hacks aren't the way I do business.

Whether it takes you 66, 100, or 250 days to create healthy habits in your life, IT WILL BE WORTH IT. Habits are such a powerful force, we often take them for granted. Once you put in the work to create empowering habit loops, your body and your mind will reap the rewards. Imagine creating a subconscious autopilot for your habits of health the way you have created the ones you possess behind the wheel of a car. No longer will you have to think long and hard about healthy food choices. Never again will you have to give yourself a pep talk every time you head off to the gym. No more conscious thought about self-talk or self-worth. You will just do the things you're supposed to do, without thinking twice about them.

Redefine your rituals. Overhaul your habits. In fitness, nutrition, and mindset, your habits will be your most powerful weapons—or your greatest weaknesses. Put in the work to progress through your patterns. You are absolutely worth it.

Testimonials from the Thrive Tribe

Meet Keith R.:

I just want to say that I have been down the road of fitness and health many times. At times in my life, I have been in great shape, but there were also times where I definitely wasn't. Inconsistency has become a theme in my journey to health and fitness. The real "light bulb" moment for me came when I heard Jay Nixon tell us to "fall in love with the process and not the prize." I really sat back and reflected on that idea, and it has made a major impact on my entire life. I have used this idea in every area of my life, not just weight loss. I am so thankful that I heard him refer to this idea very early in the process, and I have held onto it ever since. I have fallen in love with each habit, ritual, and part of the process that has ultimately shaped my health.

Jay's Journal

We are our rituals. What we do consistently day in and day out defines us. Today and every day I will audit my rituals, ensuring that my daily habits move me closer to being my best self.

Your Journal

_____

_____

_____

_____

Actions to Overcome the Overweight Mind

POWER Action Step: Incorporate the Thrive Three into your morning routine. As a quick refresher, the Thrive Three consists of writing down three things you're grateful for; writing down three things you will take positive action on during the day; and giving three high fives, hugs, or messages of encouragement to people in your life. Trust me, it will set an amazing foundation for your day.

Three Things You're Grateful For	Three Positive Action Steps	Three People You're Going To Encourage
1)	1)	1)
2)	2)	2)
3)	3)	3)

SUPER Action Step: I want you to try to identify one bad habit loop for yourself. Treat yourself like a science experiment. If you know you have a bad habit of rolling through the drive-thru after work every day, investigate and note the cue, the routine, and the reward. Keep a log of how you feel throughout the process and see how you can change it using advice given in this chapter.

BONUS Action Step: Start taking in 30 grams of quality protein every morning. I recommend consuming this in the form of a protein shake. The benefits of a quick and easy protein shake outweigh that of a bowl of cereal or donut immensely.

Chapter 3

Eater's Remorse

The first wealth is health.

–Ralph Waldo Emerson

Glennon Doyle Melton, author of *Love Warrior*, refers to food, alcohol, and other vices she encountered in her life as "easy buttons." They were things she used to numb some sort of pain, to distract her from discomfort, and to push away feelings she wanted to avoid.

What are your easy buttons? Alcohol? Chocolate? The coffee that feels healthy but is actually 300+ calories? Almost everyone has them. You feel something—stress, discomfort, or sadness—and you reach for the closest pacifier. It's a temporary fix to your immediate emotional needs, but these Band-Aid fixes to your emotional state can snowball into plenty of damage to your physical body.

Stop feeding your feelings and starting feeding your body. This is going to take tremendous awareness on your part, which will take time and practice. Awareness is like a muscle; it only grows when you intentionally use it. The next time you find yourself elbow deep in a bag of chips, stop and ask yourself why you're throwing down chips by the handful. Is it because they taste good? Possibly. Is it because they're good for you? Not a chance. Is it because you've had a rough day and eating the chips gives you a small feeling of controlled happiness?

Now you're onto something. You see, awareness can't be faked. If you can't be honest with yourself about why you're eating what you're eating, you'll be more and more likely to continue to push those "easy buttons."

On top of being honest with yourself in the short term, take a minute and consider the long term. In the movie *Austin Powers: The Spy Who Shagged Me,* the character known as Fat Bastard sums up the long game pretty well:

"I can't stop eating. I eat because I'm unhappy, and I'm unhappy because I eat. It's a vicious cycle."

Sadly, Fat Bastard has a point. It *is* a vicious cycle, and it's one imprisoning many of my clients. Some event gives them an emotional reaction. Their subconscious mind leads them right back to the fridge for a binge-eating session. Then, they wake up in the morning, think about all the things they ate and drank the day before, and inevitably sink deeper into the same sadness or stress that started the process in the first place. The eating, drinking, and repetitive pressing of these "easy buttons" only make the problems worse. To silence the exacerbated feelings of sadness, stress, or failure, they reach for the closest pacifier they hope will make them feel better. And so it goes, on and on and on.

> *Food is fuel and not a solution to anything other than giving*
> *your body nutrients. I love chocolate like the next girl, but it's*
> *not going to change my situation.*
> –Gabrielle Reece

If you've ever experienced buyer's remorse, you probably know the feeling of regret and anguish many of my clients felt. Buyer's remorse usually stems from the purchase of something big and expensive: a house, a car, or anything else worth thousands of dollars. After the purchase is made, the buyer quickly feels a sense of regret due to the extravagant spending. Thoughts like, "Did I spend too much?" and "I shouldn't have done that" swirl around in their heads, causing anxiety and sometimes depression. Buying a house or a car is a major life decision for most, and with it comes tremendous pressure. If someone feels they haven't made the right decision, they can face an ugly downward spiral of negative emotion. I like to think of Fat Bastard's vicious cycle as eater's remorse. You eat something you shouldn't have, so you pile unhealthy emotions on top of the unhealthy food choice. The emotions you attach to your food choices put you in a bad psychological space, causing you to reach for pacifiers—more unhealthy food choices—that will temporarily numb the sadness or stress of the original decision. But, as the temporary fix fades, and you realize you did it again, your emotional state sags.

How do you avoid eater's remorse and break the vicious cycle? Think back to our last chapter about habits. Focus on the cues or triggers that cause you to reach for a cinnamon roll or brownie. Of course, you eventually want to replace the action of making unhealthy food choices, but first you need to be aware of *why* you're eating something.

Are you seeking comfort? Are you hoping to replace an absence of love and connection in your life with an indulgence of ice cream, chocolate, or wine? Are you snuffing out stress with something sweet? No matter the unhealthy nutrition choices, I promise you there is a bigger reason behind them than taste or texture.

Tony Robbins speaks at length in his seminars and books about the six core human needs: Certainty, Uncertainty/Variety, Significance, Love/Connection, Growth, and Contribution. I'd be willing to guess you are trying to fill a gaping hole in one of these needs with any indulgence and fatty food escape.

Under the umbrella of certainty lies comfort. There's a reason *comfort food* is a thing. Food can often be a place where we seek comfort when life, our relationships, or our jobs aren't offering any.

The need for love and connection is so powerful that the absence of it can open up the opportunity for a loving connection with unhealthy food. Any movie storyline involving a big break-up often leads to one or both parties reaching for a tub of ice cream or a glass of wine. This is such a popular way to tell the story of a couple parting ways because it's real and happens to *a lot* of people. Love and connection may be the strongest of all human needs. When it's ripped away from us, we need a pacifier. It isn't surprising we turn to food or drink to provide comfort or numbness.

What you are attempting to suppress is not primary. Tune into the emotions and needs driving your craving—be aware of them. Once you recognize them, you can begin to shift your mindset or your actions to create a more positive way to cope.

Keeping a food journal helps—a lot! You've probably seen many health gurus advising clients to keep food journals. My focus differs a little. Most food journal advocates simply want you to write down what you eat in order to raise awareness of your caloric intake, food quality, etc. You know what that sounds like? Mechanics. Tracking your food intake and your calorie count is all mechanics. It's a piece of the puzzle, but nowhere close to the entire picture.

How is my approach different? I want you to keep track of what you eat, then *write a sentence or two* about how you were *feeling* before you decided to chow down. The simple act of recording will make the connection between emotions and eating concrete and demonstrate your emotional state in relation to food choices. Over the course of a week (or a month), you will begin to spot your triggers and cues very plainly. Increased awareness will enable you to experiment with changing your emotional eating habits.

Something to note here: this journal is NOT a forum for you to judge yourself. You need to write your pre-eating thoughts and feelings as honestly as possible. Then you can look at your information and find ways to change. If you claim you felt happy before you took a trip to McDonald's, chances are you're not being genuine. The point of the journal is to open an objective window into your mind. Once you collect enough entries, the patterns you once considered a mystery will show themselves with clarity. You will never again ask, "Why do I keep eating this crap?" The answers will stare you in the face.

Remember, to make big changes in your health and fitness, our focus is 80% psychology and 20% mechanics. Your emotions take up a lot of space and it's important for you see to them clearly and honestly. It doesn't matter how many miles you run or burpees you do if your emotions have a stranglehold on your food choices.

Feed your body and not your feelings. You'll be *happy* you did.

Testimonials from the Thrive Tribe

Meet JC Rod:

As I stood on the scale, I saw the number that I told myself I would never weigh. I stared at that 300 pound number and told myself, "That's it! It's time to eat healthy and workout! But first, one last trip to the buffet before I eat clean."

After the buffet, it was, "Well, now I need to have pizza one last time." Than I had to have burgers and fries one last time.

Then when the scale showed "305" I told myself, "310 is a strong and even number. I will get serious about my health when I hit that number." So then my cycle of eating bad food continued. When I hit 310, I gave myself the excuse to start when I reach 315. I allowed myself to use excuse after excuse. I was allowing myself to continue to fail and abuse my body.

My fiancée was in Jay's program and had lost 50 pounds. I had seen the success her boss was having as well. I was scared to join the program because I had the evidence that his program obviously worked and if I didn't lose the weight, it was all on me. I wouldn't have an excuse to blame it on the program. My success rested solely on my shoulders.

After much hesitation and being done with allowing myself to use excuse after excuse, I finally joined Jay's program. Best decision I ever made (besides asking my fiancée to marry me!). After four months in Jay's program, I am in the best shape of my life!

Jay's Journal

Planning my meals is the key to my success. When I'm intentional in my decisions to eat healthy, nutritious foods, my success is predictable. Today I will eat the foods I've planned and prepared. I will not allow my emotions or the events of the day to derail my plan for nutritional success. There will be no surprises in my eating today. Planning = success.

Your Journal

_____

_____

_____

_____

_____

_____

Actions to Overcome the Overweight Mind

POWER Action Step: Identify three emotional triggers. Write them down. Look for them. Pay attention to them. Your emotions may not change, but your response to them surely can. You may eat fast food only after you get stressed out at work. You may only eat chocolate when you're sad. Figure out your emotional triggers and put them on paper.

Emotional Triggers
Work Stress

SUPER Action Step: Okay, you've figured out your emotional triggers. Brainstorm replacement actions you can introduce. Instead of resorting to fast food for work stress, keep a pack of gum in your car so you have something to chew. When you're feeling sad, replace a chocolate bar with a chocolate protein shake. Write down different ways you can combat your emotional triggers.

Emotional Trigger	Current Action	New Action
1) Work Stress	Open a bottle of wine	Get outside for a family walk
2)		
3)		
4)		

Chapter 4

....

Three Things More Important to Track than Fats, Carbs, and Protein: Beliefs, Thoughts, and Words

Your beliefs become your thoughts, your thoughts become your words, your words become your actions, your actions become your habits, your habits become your values, your values become your destiny.

–Mahatma Gandhi

Gandhi's quotation outlines the essence of this book. Start with your beliefs and arrive at your destiny. I am less concerned with surface-level fixes and more interested in deep, powerful lifestyle shifts. I can prescribe a restrictive diet, an exhaustive workout plan, and throw multiple other quick-fix gimmicks your way, but they won't create lasting change to your health. A lot of things will probably work in the short term, but without seismic shifts, you'll be right back where you started in time.

Remember our friends from *The Biggest Loser*? Starvation tactics, crazy workout regimens, and a lack of mindset work built a weak foundation for their lifelong health. Most of the contestants we discussed gained all of their weight back within five years of the show. It seems like they only read the last half of Gandhi's quotation before they got to work. They focused more on the *action*, and forgot to address their beliefs, thoughts, and words. I won't do you such a disservice.

1. What do you *believe* you're capable of doing?

2. What do you *think* of yourself?

3. What *words* do you use to describe your goals, your dreams, and your life?

Those three questions will make or break your fitness journey. Guaranteed.

Beliefs

What do you believe you are capable of achieving? So many of my clients come to me because they have tried other trainers, programs, or diets and haven't found success. By the time they get to me, how many believe that they can actually lose the weight they want? Not many at all. They hope I can give them some magic workout or meal plan to solve all of their problems. If I tried to sell them on that magic plan, I'd be dishonest in the attempt. It doesn't exist. Instead, I throw all of the mechanics out the window and address their beliefs. If they don't believe they can do it, they are wasting their time and their money.

Taking care of your belief system will take you longer than a 30–60 minute workout, but the results will ripple through all areas of your life. You *need* to believe in your goals. You *need* to believe in your worth. You *need* to believe in yourself.

Beliefs are often based in truth. The reason some of my clients don't believe they can lose their desired weight when they meet me is because they've spent years trying with little success. They have a backlog of evidence screaming, "You can't do this."

How do you turn the tide of negative evidence? You immerse yourself in stories of incredible weight loss. You surround yourself with people who have the same goals as you—people who have actually accomplished them. You surround yourself with positive messaging that inspires you. In order to overcome the mounting evidence of failure from your past, you need to pile on evidence of success—evidence of what is possible—to create a beautiful foundation for your future.

The story of Roger Bannister may be overplayed by now, but it's worth mentioning when it comes to breaking false beliefs. In 1954, Bannister ran a mile in under four minutes, the first time anyone had ever done so officially. In the years leading up to his historic run, the record for the fastest mile sat for nine years at 4:01.4. Prior to the mark of 4:01.4, the world record in the mile run fell by a second or two every year. But, as the record inched towards four minutes, progress slowed.

Why did it take so long for someone to run the mile in under four minutes? The same reason you can't seem to keep the weight off, get your butt out of bed to hit the gym, or stop picking at the donut spread at work: it *seems* impossible. A time below 4:00.0 sounded like a fictional narrative to the runners of that time. "It's never been done before, so what suggests it can be done now?" they thought. Insert Bannister and his conquering of the four-minute barrier.

Want to know what happened after Roger Bannister clocked a time of 3:59.4? Once runners saw the intimidating plateau could be broken, the impossible became possible. By the end of that year, another man, John Landy, ran the mile in 3:58.0. A handful of other men ran sub-four-minute miles in 1955 and 1956 as well. Within ten years, Bannister's monumental 3:59.4 had been trimmed by five seconds down to 3:54.1. All it took was one man to show everyone that what was once considered impossible was, in fact, possible. Psychological barriers can be just as intimidating as physical ones.

Your beliefs matter. If you don't believe you can create positive change in your life, find ways to witness what your brain deems impossible. There are people who have already done what you want to accomplish. Find them and use their stories as inspiration. If another human being has pulled off what you want, I bet you can find a way to do the same.

Thoughts

Whether you think you can or you think you can't – you're right.

–Henry Ford

It's as simple as Ford suggests. At the beginning of the chapter, Gandhi suggests your thoughts will eventually lead to your destiny. Ford's point is that if you begin with negative beliefs (which will translate into negative thoughts), what do you think your destiny will look like?

That's not really a rhetorical question. Where do you think your negative thoughts will take you? Nowhere pleasant, I'm sure. It's time you reframe your thoughts and emotions and point them in a positive direction. You can't control many of life's circumstances, but you *can* control how you think about them.

I like to look at opportunity versus obligation. Do you feel grateful for the *opportunity* to exercise and to move your body, or do you resent your workout? Do you love the chance to nourish your body with quality food, or do you think, "This broccoli insults my taste buds"? Whatever the external event, you get to choose your attitude towards it. By shifting your thoughts from a place of obligation to one of opportunity, your thoughts will breathe positivity into the rest of your life.

You won't resent your weight-loss journey anymore because you will see the opportunity for a healthy, vibrant life. The early mornings won't be a chore because you will understand that you are setting a strong foundation for your day.

You might experience the same day as everyone else, but you can think about the events in a completely different way. Your thoughts—how you view your daily routine—change everything. They permeate positive or negative results through the rest of your life. Be aware of your thoughts. Opportunity serves you, while obligation leaves you resenting your every move. Choose wisely.

There are three specific thought patterns I observe in my clients and people in general that stunt their growth as they pursue whatever goals they've set. These persisting thoughts are poisonous in health, business, relationships, and life in general, so let's take a little time dispelling them.

"I Don't Have Time"

Wrong. You have plenty of time, just poor time *management*. At the very least, you're choosing not to make time for what's important. You've found time for Netflix, happy hour, or movie night, but you just can't seem to find the time for an hour of exercise. Odd that you can't rearrange a few things. If you want a healthy lifestyle badly enough, you can shift your schedule around to make things work.

There are numerous examples of people who have kids, jobs, and other obligations who still manage to keep themselves in shape. I can help break apart the "not enough time" issue with almost all of my clients. They only *thought* they didn't have time to exercise or plan their meals, but I teach them how to prioritize their 24 hours to their optimum advantage.

- » 10 hours for work
- » 8 hours for sleep
- » 4 hours for family
- » 1 hour for "me time"

Even with these generous allocations of time, there's still 1 hour left for exercise. You don't even need an entire hour; 30 minutes of hard work will do just fine. The point is this: thinking you don't have time is completely false. You can always make the time; you just need to adjust your priorities.

"I Don't Know How"

There may be some truth here, but it shouldn't be a permanent fixture in your mind. Life is a constant learning process. Every day presents the chance to convert "I don't know how" into "Now I understand." Do you think I knew everything there was to know about coaching, fitness, and nutrition when I began my business? Not a chance. I knew a fair amount from studying health and business, but the difference between what I know now and what I knew then is *massive*.

You can't let your lack of knowledge hold you back. Once you acknowledge your lack of experience, you can use the truth to move forward. You can become intentional about learning something new.

Find a coach, a trainer, or a mentor—someone who can help you convert your "I don't know" into "Now I understand." You can always find resources—people, books, or courses—to help you bridge the knowledge gap.

"I Don't Know Where to Start"

No kidding! No one expects you to know where to start. If you have a goal and know every step required to achieve it, you would've done it already. It's okay to be a novice or an amateur because there are always professionals who can help you. They've been there before and can assist you to find an appropriate starting point. The finish line is always a clear image in your mind, but if you can't find the starting line, the finish line doesn't matter. Find a professional (like me) to guide you towards the right path and see you through to the finish line.

Thoughts can either be powerful or leave you powerless. But you choose your thoughts. Whenever a thought passes through your mind, decide if it's serving you or not, then use or dismiss accordingly.

Words

Let's observe the same situation from the perspective of two different people. It could be a married couple, best friends, or coworkers—you choose. Whatever the case, each person has the same plans tomorrow morning: waking up early to get a workout in before heading off to work.

Person #1: "Tomorrow morning I have to get up at 4:30 a.m. to do my workout. If I wait until after work, I'll have to fight rush hour traffic and a crowded gym just to get some decent exercise. Once I finish my workout, it's time to ship off for an eight-hour shift. I wish I could get an IV of coffee upon arrival."

Person #2: "Tomorrow morning I get to wake up nice and early and start my day off with a challenging and invigorating workout. Sure, I'm getting up at 4:30 a.m., but it's a great way to start the day and gives me the energy I need to be productive at work. It may be early, but I can't think of a better way to start my day with more positive momentum."

Same situation, two different perspectives. Who do you think is going to have a better workout? Who do you think is going to have a better day at work? Who do you think is going to have a better day overall? That's right, Person #2 in a unanimous decision.

Why?

The words you use matter immensely. Everything you say dresses your day in positivity or negativity. Person #2 chooses to say he "gets to arise early" and start his day off with an early morning workout. Person #1 opts for "I *have* to get up at 4:30 a.m. just to do my workout." Subtle differences like "I get to" versus "I have to" can make a substantial difference in your actions. "I get to" breathes gratitude and opportunity into your early morning workout. If you "get to" workout, you're thankful for the privilege to move your body around. If you "have to" get up early and workout, it feels more like a chore or punishment.

Your vocabulary rests somewhere on a spectrum. At one end of the spectrum you have words with negative, limiting connotations. Words and phrases like "I can't," "impossible," and "I have to" hang out on that end. On the other end of the spectrum are words that project positivity. Phrases like "I am," "I will," and "Yes!" anchor this side of the spectrum. No matter where you find yourself, there's always room to improve. I truly believe the vocabulary you use can transform your attitude, your actions, and your life.

Discard phrases like "I can't do..." and replace them with "I'm currently working on..." When you let negative phrases ooze out of your mouth, your mind has already decided between success and failure, and the results are not in your favor. By shifting your words and phrasing from the negative end of the spectrum to the positive end, your mind gets a head start towards success. Small changes in your vocabulary will transform your health, fitness, and life. I promise.

Want to know another word I hate? "Diet." That hurt just writing it.

You'll never hear me say that word to any of my clients. The word itself isn't bad, but the connotation our culture has put on it decreases its value. By definition, a "diet" is simply the food you habitually eat. "Diet" has morphed into a fast-tracked weight-loss, food-deprivation, starvation "program."

"Diet" in this sense also always comes with an end date. If someone tells you that they're going on a diet, it's likely some ten- to twelve-week program with an end goal similar to a vacation, wedding, or some other big event. They'll eat less, lose the weight, cross the finish line, then return to what they were previously doing.

I'm not in the business of quick fixes or weight-loss goals that don't stick. That's why I don't like to use the word "diet" with my Tribe. My goal is to make weight loss and health goals last for a lifetime. I deliver a lifestyle, not a get-thin-quick scheme. Diet has no place in my world. Figure out what words have no place in your world. What words aren't serving you at all? Either discard them or replace them with something more positive. Your words are your choice. Choose something that paints a positive picture for you on a daily basis.

Again, your awareness stands at the forefront of making a positive shift here. You can't change bad habits unless you're aware of them. You can't stop your emotional eating until you're aware of those emotions and their effect on your food consumption. Similarly, you can't change your beliefs, thoughts, or words without being aware of where you currently stand with them. Be more conscious of your thoughts throughout the day. Take note of the words you're using. You can't make a change until you see a problem for what it is.

Your beliefs, your thoughts, and your words are all in your power. Every day, you get to decide how they impact your progress in health, in fitness, and in life. The more you open your eyes to how you're currently using these three things, the easier it will be to shift them all for the better. Be honest with yourself and start creating the destiny you deserve.

I *believe* you. I *think* you are more capable than you think you are. I am *telling* you, whatever your goal, you have the ability to crush it.

Testimonials from the Thrive Tribe

Meet Joe and Stacy M.:

We never thought that trying to drop a few pounds would forever change our marriage. Our small story turns into an epic journey with a lucky draw and a winning ticket.

Over the course of our first six-week challenge with Jay, we found a common goal and began to collaborate on meal planning, workouts and a healthier way to raise our son. Six weeks turned into 12 weeks, 12 turned into 24, and so on. As time went on, our household centered on Jay's weekly check-ins with the Tribe and his positive messaging. As our new normal set in, it opened a deeper dialog between us as husband and wife. We began looking for every opportunity to motivate each other in everything. Jay is a daily and sometimes hourly reminder that our big aspirations will materialize, removing the fear and assuring us we deserve to achieve big. "You can be, do and have anything you want!" For the first time in our life, we truly believe it.

This is a hard-working drive we are instilling in our son early. Our whole family is on a path for greatness and it is simply because we were blessed enough to cross paths with Jay. He has been there when we falter, with no judgment and just the right words. We now know our "After" picture is just the beginning of our epic journey that began with putting one foot in front of the other.

Jay's Journal

Today my thoughts and my words will be positive and purposeful. Staying aware of my thoughts, words, and actions will allow me to focus on my goals. Keep the main thing the main thing.

Your Journal

_____

_____

_____

Actions to Overcome the Overweight Mind

POWER Action Step: Identify one limiting belief you have about yourself. It might be something like "I'm not good enough" or "I don't deserve this." Once you've identified your limiting and negative belief, write down how to convert the thought into something positive.

Example: "I don't deserve to lose the weight" becomes "I DO deserve to lose this weight." If you look hard enough, there will always be evidence to prove your limiting belief wrong. Discover that evidence and unlock the restraints holding you back.

SUPER Action Step: For the next week, wear a rubber band on your wrist. Every time you use a word that doesn't serve your goals (i.e. "I can't," "I won't," "I have to"), snap the rubber band on your wrist. Sure it's a small, stinging pain, but it will serve as a negative connection for your brain. Your brain knows touching a pan on a hot stove is not good, so it knows not to do it. By snapping a rubber band on your wrist every time you let a negative word fly, your brain will allow fewer and fewer of them. The negative correlation between pain and negative words will ensure reduced, ever-decreasing use.

Chapter 5

Standards – Raise the Bar

If you want to change your life, you have to change your standards.

–Tony Robbins

You get what you tolerate. In your career, in your relationships, and in your health, *you get what you tolerate.* Your standards are yours to choose. You decide what is acceptable or unacceptable. Still, not many people consciously choose their standards. They wander through life, not too particular about their expectations, and eventually they end up dissatisfied. This is such a backwards approach. You cannot anticipate great results on the backend if you haven't set clear and high standards on the front end. By taking the time to decide exactly what you'll allow, you have a distinct moral compass guiding you through daily subconscious decisions.

Maybe you haven't set your standards high enough. Maybe it's been a long time since you even considered what you will tolerate in your life. That's probably why you picked up this book in the first place. You want to make a change. You want to see a difference in your health and fitness. One of the biggest steps you can take is raising your standards. Raise your standard of nutrition. Raise your standard of exercise. Raise your standard of living. Know your worth and set the bar accordingly.

How high is too high? How worthy are you? It may seem difficult to assess, but you'll know it when you see it. Standards are absolutes. Something is either acceptable, or it's not. Often, the best way to identify what you *will* allow in your life is by recognizing what you absolutely *won't*.

An area of our life that showcases our standards in plain sight is our relationships. You can observe someone's marriage or a young courtship and see exactly what those two people allow. We've all had a friend come to us and say something like, "I don't know why they keep cheating on me!" I'm sorry…keep? That would indicate your friend has known about the infidelity, acknowledged it, and has come to accept it as appropriate behavior.

Apparently, they find cheating acceptable. By setting the bar so low, they've opened themselves to disappointment. They're not allowed to be unhappy about an unfaithful partner if they're allowing it to happen.

For most of us, our first thought is, "Oh no, that wouldn't fly with me." You know your own standard. By knowing exactly what you won't allow, you shine a light on what you will. While your friend may be naively allowing an unfaithful partner to step out, you know you won't. Put more positively, you mandate fidelity!

You have established your bar.

Using relationships as a tool to paint the picture of standards is useful because everyone can relate. You know what is acceptable, and I'd assume your partner does as well. It's set in stone, and anyone who isn't up to the task of meeting your standards won't be around for long. Think about some of your failed relationships. Most of us have quite a few. When those relationships were finally over, it gave you time to reflect on what worked (not much) and what didn't (plenty). Right then and there, you decided to raise your standards.

"I'll never let that happen again."

"I won't ever accept being treated like that in the future."

Right?

"Never again," you said.

Now, let's look at the most important relationship in your life: the one with yourself. Are your standards with yourself as clear as they are with others? Do you know, without fail, exactly what is acceptable or unacceptable? Your health and fitness are a large part of this relationship. By taking care of your body, you're professing self-love. By taking in high-quality food, you're nourishing yourself. You're showing yourself respect. You're showing you care about yourself.

You have established your bar.

If your overall health has slipped, it's because you've allowed it. Your standards and expectations for your well-being have been lowered enough for all bad habits to persist. Like your friend who turned a blind eye to their cheating partner, you've looked the other way with regard to your late-night snacking and vague commitment to exercise.

> *You teach people how to treat you by what you allow,*
> *what you stop, and what you reinforce.*
>
> –Tony Gaskins

It's time you raised your standards.

In relationships, your partner's commitment isn't just suggested; it's mandatory. You need to have the same standard of commitment to yourself. Have the same respect for yourself you would demand from others. I don't want to hear you say, "I should probably lose some weight." That won't get you anywhere. Use, "I must lose 20 pounds." Set the standard high. It's non-negotiable. Don't give yourself a loophole to back out at a later date. Turn all of your "shoulds" into "musts." Make your standards mandatory.

You've already found your "why." Let your "why" be the driving force in crafting your new standards. Whether it's playing with your grandkids, feeling alive again, or rekindling your stagnant relationship, your "why" will keep your standards strong. It will put real meaning behind what is acceptable and unacceptable within your healthy lifestyle.

When you reach for a cookie, your first conscious thought may be, "Unacceptable by my standards." As much as I'd love to say that will ward off all cookie binges, it won't. What *will* help is a powerful "why" holding your standards in place. You won't shrug off the cookie and say, "One cookie won't kill me." You'll remember that the reason you're trying to live a healthy lifestyle is to *make sure* the cookies don't kill you. You want to live long enough to see your kids get married and watch your grandkids grow. Even though it's only one cookie, it's not worth messing with your ultimate goal.

So, what have we learned so far?

» You need to raise your standards of health and fitness in order to attain sustained success moving forward.

» Tolerate less and demand more of yourself.

» Remember your "why" to set your standards in stone. Your "why" will give those standards and expectations meaningful conviction each and every day.

I want to warn you about what happens when you begin to see amazing results. You'll eventually meet your goals and surpass your limits.

What happens then? Self-sabotage.

In his book, *The Big Leap*, Gay Hendricks goes into detail about what happens when you reach your upper limit, the edge of your comfort zone. We've felt the unnerving vulnerability of stepping over the edge of our comfort zone. Surpassing your upper limit is essentially stepping over a comfortable line of success.

Whether a weight-loss goal, a promotion at work, or landing someone who you think is out of your league, there's a subconscious line you feel you're not worthy of crossing. Hendricks suggests when people surpass their upper limit, it makes them uncomfortable. So uncomfortable, in fact, it's not uncommon to see people self-sabotage to bring them back to a state of normalcy. If you find yourself reaching and surpassing your upper limits, understand you *are* worthy of what you achieved. You're going to be on a well-deserved high from your accomplishments, but by surpassing your upper limit, you may subconsciously trigger a desire to come back down to earth.

Don't you dare come down. Don't convince yourself you don't deserve your best body and mind. Keep your standards high and your excuses low. Raise the bar for your life and understand it's necessary to your progress. You won't be able to lose the weight until you determine it is unacceptable not to lose it. You won't be able to keep the weight off until it's mandatory that you do. Expect more from yourself and know you deserve every bit of the "more" you create.

Testimonials from the Thrive Tribe:

Meet Laurilie J.:

I am 46 years old, a mother of three girls, ages 16, 15, and 11, and I work as a media instructor at a community college in Palm Desert, California. I am a former news anchor and reporter so my appearance was everything. Over the past decade our family went through some tough times. I had a blood clot in my leg after childbirth that put me on bed rest for months, I lost my father who suffered for nine months with a painful cancer, and we packed and moved several times. I worried about everything. Stress zapped me. I gained 40 pounds and felt horrible. I knew something had to change in order to be an active, healthy mother and a positive example to my girls. I tried everything from Jenny Craig to Weight Watchers to Medifast. Sure, I saw some short-term results, but no diet gave me the right tools for success. After a recent summer vacation with my family, I came home feeling depressed. What next?

Some friends had been talking about this program called Thrive with Jay Nixon. I met with Jay and started immediately. Jay's passion, positive attitude, support, and encouragement have inspired me to be my best. I was nervous about the accountability and the intense workouts, but soon realized these things were exactly what I needed. There is no easy fix. Jay's weekly Q & A calls prepared me mentally for every stage of this journey. I have been on the program for four months, I have lost 34 pounds, I am stronger, more confident, and mentally I know I can achieve anything. My body shape has completely changed. This is a lifelong journey and I couldn't be happier. No more fads, quick fixes, or gimmicks. Jay taught me how to raise my standards and to realize I deserved more. I have learned eating right, exercise, a healthy mental state, accountability, and Jay's wisdom are the reasons for my success. My family is proud, my friends are proud and I am proud of the new me. Thanks Jay and the entire Tribe for helping me become my best!

Jay's Journal

I am my standards. How I treat myself matters and teaches others how to treat me. Today, I will raise my standards to a new level of excellence.

Your Journal

_____

_____

_____

_____

_____

_____

Actions to Overcome the Overweight Mind

POWER Action Step: It's time to stop thinking about raising your standards and put some action towards actually doing it. Below are three spaces where you will turn three "shoulds" into three "musts."

Whatever your goals are, they will be more easily achieved with more certainty in your standards. These statements could be about your fitness level, the quality of your nutrition, or anything else having to do with your goal of living a healthier lifestyle. Be intentional about this exercise, as if you were writing a legal contract with yourself. Once you've written down these three "musts," you will know what MUST be done moving forward.

Here's an example to get the juices flowing:

Should: I should hit the gym three times a week.

Must: I must hit the gym three times a week.

A simple shift, but the word "must" is absolute. There's no wiggle room or loopholes here. It's your turn. Create the "musts" that will change your life below:

This is all a **POWER Action Step**, so it's non-negotiable. Do the work to create change in your life.

Should #1:

_____

_____

Must #1:

_____

_____

Should #2:

_____

_____

Must #2:

_____

_____

Should #3:

_____

_____

Must #3:

_____

_____

Feel that? That's the standard of your life being raised. Since YOU created these changes, the ownership in these decisions is all yours. If you fail to meet these new standards, you're not letting me down; it's you that you're going to disappoint.

SUPER Action Step: As you grow, your "musts" should grow. At the end of every month, evaluate your "musts" and make sure they are constantly evolving.

Chapter 6

....

Circle of Success

You are the average of the five people you spend the most time with.

–Jim Rohn

DeMarco Murray was the talk of the National Football League in 2014. In just his fourth season in the league, all with the Dallas Cowboys, he led all running backs with 1,845 rushing yards and was ahead of the second leading rusher by nearly 500 yards.

Things were looking up for Murray. He hit his stride at just the right time; 2014 was the last year of his contract. Translation: he'd set himself up for quite the payday. He was about to become the belle of the free agent ball. He was now available to entertain contracts from any and every team in the NFL. Any team lacking in the running back department drew up a contract and sent it his way. After such an incredible season, he had plenty of suitors willing to pay him $8–$10 million a year to repeat his success.

When the dust settled from the bidding war for Murray, it was the Philadelphia Eagles—one of his former team's rivals—that secured DeMarco and his impressive running abilities. He would be joining an Eagles offense many thought would be dynamic. Head Coach Chip Kelly, former University of Oregon coach and offensive guru, stood at the helm. Kelly was known for his fast-paced offensive schemes, and football fans across the country were excited to see what he could do with the explosive talent of Murray.

So how'd it go? Murray stormed on the scene in Philadelphia and racked up a whopping…702 rushing yards in 2015.

Well, he must've gotten hurt, right?

No, not at all. In 2014, his breakout year of 1,845 rushing yards with the Cowboys, he played in all 16 games. In 2015, that first year with the Eagles, he played in 15. His playing time was essentially the same as the year before, but his rushing totals decreased by half…and then some.

So, what was it? What I haven't mentioned to this point is what some suggest was the cause of Murray's ascent and subsequent fall from grace: the Dallas Cowboys offensive line. During the 2014 season, the Cowboys offensive line was widely considered the best in the business. Offensive linemen essentially have two jobs: protecting the quarterback and pushing the defense around so the running back can break free. The five 300+-pound men wearing Cowboys' uniforms each week performed their tasks at a consistently high level.

While running behind this offensive line, Murray's job was a little easier. Sure, he was a talented player, but having the "big uglies" in front of him increased his rate of success. They literally paved the way for him to do what he does best, opening up space for him to run week after week. When he left Dallas, he left those five men in the process. When he arrived in Philadelphia, he had less help around him, less support to lean on, and his numbers dropped significantly. He was the same player, but by leaving the support system he had in Dallas, his productivity screeched to a halt. What seemed to be a bright future in Philly turned dark quickly.

Contrast DeMarco Murray's story with that of LeBron James. Upon his arrival to the National Basketball Association, James spent seven seasons with his hometown Cleveland Cavaliers. He was one of the most physically talented players in the league during those seven seasons, winning the MVP award in two of them. His skills and show-manship drew comparisons to all-time greats like Michael Jordan and Magic Johnson, but he knew he wouldn't reach true upper echelon status until he could win a title. As hard as he worked and despite his skill level, he couldn't bring home a championship. Year after year he and the Cavs would impress in the regular season, then falter in the playoffs.

After the highs and lows of those initial seasons with the Cavaliers, LeBron signed as a free agent with the Miami Heat, joining forces with fellow superstars Dwyane Wade and Chris Bosh. Wade already had a championship ring, and Bosh was an up-and-coming talent in the NBA. James spent four years in Miami, reaching the NBA Finals in all four. In two of those trips to the Finals, he exited with the honor of Finals MVP and a championship ring.

What changed? What was different? He had been a great player prior to his time with Miami. While in Cleveland, he was a two-time Most Valuable Player. The notable difference wasn't LeBron at all; it was the players surrounding him. They were talented for sure, but, more important, they were seasoned. They knew what it took to win. They had the work ethic to get it done. In Cleveland he was a solo artist, but in Miami he was part of a harmonious group.

These stories illustrate how powerful it is to surround yourself with a Circle of Success. I use these athletes' experiences because, in sports, there are metrics to show notable progression or regression. In the case of LeBron James, he was able to secure two league championships in his Circle of Success. DeMarco Murray saw his productivity slip by more than 50% once he walked away from his.

Find yourself a Circle of Success. If you can't find one, create one. Few things create a more powerful and positive change than getting around people who share the same attitudes, beliefs, and goals as you.

I am proud to be a part of the Thrive Tribe, my Circle of Success. I'd love to take credit for its incredible culture, but I'm only one of many who have helped build it. It's amazing to see the safe and supportive space within the Tribe. It has been a place where people with little to no fitness experience have cultivated a healthy lifestyle and transformed their daily lives. Sure, I may lead the pack, but we all help each other grow and get better each and every day. Having a group of like-minded people around you is a priceless asset.

Make a conscious effort to surround yourself with positive, nourishing, and uplifting people— people who believe in you, encourage you to go after your dreams, and applaud your victories.

–Jack Canfield

Let your mind wander for a minute, here. Think about the times you've tried to lose some weight or improve your nutrition. (Maybe that time is now.) You woke up one day and decided you were going to live a healthier life. Now consider the people closest to you and the effect they had on the outcome.

Let's start at home. Odds are, your spouse didn't have the same weight-loss epiphany on the same night that you did. It's hard to get your partner to hop on the healthy bandwagon, no matter how much he/she loves you. It's hard enough changing your habits; good luck changing someone else's.

Over time, your partner may tempt you away from your healthy habits intentionally or unintentionally. If you lose some weight, they greet your success with a supportive celebratory dinner or a reassuring "you've earned yourself some ice cream for all of your hard work." Little by little, these small, well-intentioned rewards steer you off course and lead you right back into your old comfort zone. Sooner or later, the fire inside to create lasting healthy habits is extinguished. You're right back where you started.

Now, let's take a look at your social circle. Over the years, you've grown close to your friends. You've created an image of yourself. This image generates certain expectations they have of you. If you woke up one day and decided you were no longer going to abide by those expectations, your friends might not be accepting.

If you stop going to happy hour and start hitting the gym after work, you change the dynamics of your relationships. If you quit eating pizza and drinking beer on football Sundays with your buddies, they may have some questions. They might not understand why you want to be any different from the person they know. They might think your changing is a threat to your relationship. Eventually, they'll attempt to chip away at your new habits, bit by bit. You'll get a text saying, "Come out with us tonight. It's just one night." They'll dress their requests up in guilt so you feel bad if you don't show up. "Just one night." "Just one drink." "Just one pizza." Beware of the "just one's." They'll get you every time.

I'm not suggesting you cut all ties with anyone less motivated than you.

Have a conversation with your spouse about your goals and why they mean so much to you. Make it clear why being healthy is important, but also why it serves a purpose in your relationship. Put simply, the healthier you are in body and mind, the better partner you can be to your husband or wife. If they can't appreciate that, then you have a bigger problem on your hands.

With your friends, give it time. There's going to be a period when what you're doing and how you're acting is going to make them uncomfortable. This isn't your fault. Over time, they've attached themselves to a certain idea of who you are. The moment you change your image, whether for bad or for good, it's going to rub them the wrong way. As time goes by, though, some will see you for who you really are and want to stick around. Others will continually be put off by your attempts to change. They are attached to the former person, and you can't spend your life trying to fit into the box they've created for you. It's okay to grow past some people. It's all right if you move forward and they choose to stay stagnant. You don't need their dead weight pulling you back into your old ways.

My point is this: changing your mindset and habits is going to be *extremely* difficult when everyone around you isn't moving in the same direction. Not only will it be difficult, but it's also going to be a lonely road to travel. If your friends are donut eaters, you're going to end up being a donut eater. If your spouse snacks all night long, you're going to find yourself doing the same. You need to get around people who will support and inspire you to keep growing.

Your environment needs to support your goals. The people, places, and things you immerse yourself in need to align in some way with your target. If your current support system isn't being supportive of the healthy lifestyle you'd like to lead, you need to seek out people who will.

By creating or finding a Circle of Success, your mechanics and your mindset will increase exponentially. If you come see me at my fitness studio, I am going to show what a quality workout looks like (mechanics), but also surround you with like-minded clients all working towards a healthier version of themselves (mindset). All of our workouts are done in a community format. It's never one-on-one. It's always in a large group. Why? Because when we work out together, we can feed off of each other's energy and create a positive atmosphere for our exercise. It is a living, breathing Circle of Success.

Circles of Success aren't limited to health and fitness, either. Take me, for instance. I constantly put myself in the company of like-minded individuals as I look to better myself and my business. I've participated in several mastermind groups, landing me in the same room with successful entrepreneurs looking to improve their businesses. We shared processes that worked, things that didn't, and helped each other become better at what we do best.

It's imperative to have people reminding you of your aspirations in life—directly or indirectly—every single day. More importantly, find successful people who can help guide the way.

Frank Shamrock, famed MMA fighter, has a great way to think about your Circle of Success: **Plus, Minus, Equal**. Put simply, you should have people in your Circle that are above, below, and equal to your skill set. The purpose of the plus people is obvious. They are the ones with more knowledge, skill, and experience than you. You want them around to help teach you and guide your journey to growth.

The equal ones are similar to you and your current abilities. You want them around so you can compete and compare your growth. You are on the same trajectory of change as your "equals," so you can use them as measuring sticks for your development.

The minus people are there for you to teach. As you create better habits and improve yourself, showing them the way will help ingrain your new knowledge and skills over time.

If you were to join one of my Circles of Success—the Thrive Tribe—you would be entering into a plus, minus, equal support system on day one. I would represent the plus person within the Circle, providing guidance and helping you to reach your goals. The equal representatives would be my current and former clients that are, like you, pushing themselves to change their lives. In the beginning, you would be the minus person, learning from everyone around you. As you gain experience and begin to progress, though, you would have others you could mentor and teach about your journey, leading them to a higher level.

By having all three of these elements in your Circle of Success, you will ensure your continued progress towards any goal you choose.

How do you cultivate such a Circle? How can you find the community necessary to propel you forward? Look for a fitness studio (or gym similar to mine) that emphasizes group exercise classes. By entering this community, you will immediately have people around you to support your goals and to assist you down the path of achieving them.

There are groups of people in your local community that want the same things as you. Go to meetup.com and search for people in your area with the same beliefs and goals you have created for yourself. Most of these groups are free and can put you in the same room with people who will inspire and motivate you. Just by searching "health and fitness," you will see how many people out there want what you want: a healthier lifestyle and a group of people with whom to share the mission.

If you want to take it one step further, you can invest in yourself and join a mastermind group as I have in the past. These mastermind groups cost, but by putting "skin in the game," you will quickly find you have more stock in your success. You've added the need to get your money's worth on top of your original goals. This will hold you accountable and keep your mind pushing towards and past your markers of achievement.

DeMarco Murray and LeBron James discovered that being around like-minded people with similar aspirations makes success more attainable. Do what you can to avoid years of "do it yourself," willpower-fueled ambition. It can only get you so far. If you want to lose weight, find someone who has done it and who can teach you. Find some people on the same journey and share the highs and lows along the way.

Teamwork makes the dream work. Find your team. Find your Circle of Success.

Testimonials from the Thrive Tribe

Meet Chrissy C.:

I wanted to work out with Jay to get some exercise and see my friends that were already a part of his Thrive Tribe. I have been around fitness my entire life; I am a personal trainer and Pilates instructor.

After a few months, I started to "hear" Jay. He was full of positive comments and suggestions. His Facebook posts seemed to speak only to me. His call topics were exactly what I needed to hear. I was able to connect almost everything he said and did into my life, and it had nothing to do with fitness. I had experienced a tough few years moving across the country and losing my father. I thought I was dealing with things fine. However, with Jay and the Tribe's help, I honestly felt, for the first time in my life, I was able to set realistic goals and take action. I have always set goals, don't get me wrong, but this was different. I saw myself and my life through a different perspective and it was one I was able to act on. Life is real, it's challenging, and it's totally what we make it. Jay inspired me to want to be better—and to make my mark in this world.

I am so blessed to have found Jay and to include him in my Circle of Success. I went to him for a little workout, but instead I gained inspiration, crazy motivation, and an entire new outlook on how to navigate and get the most out of this beautiful life!

I feel beyond blessed to have Jay's coaching and the Tribe in my corner—they fill a void I had no idea I had.

Jay's Journal

"We are who we hang around." Keeping this in mind as I move through my day will help me make decisions from where I want to be as opposed to where I am now. Knowing I have amazing people surrounding me keeps me centered and focused on my goal of becoming my best self.

Your Journal

_____

_____

_____

_____

_____

_____

Actions to Overcome the Overweight Mind

POWER Action Step: It's time to do some inventory on the people closest to you. Based on Jim Rohn's quote from the beginning of this chapter, I want you to write down the five people you spend the most time with, then assess their role in your success.

Step 1: Write down the five people you spend the most time with

Step 2: Fill in your three musts across the top of the table (Must #1, Must #2, Must #3 from last chapter's POWER Action Step)

Step 3: Circle a (+) or a (-) in each box to indicate if that person is a positive or negative influence on that Must.

Circle of Success Assessment	Must #1:	Must #2:	Must #3:
Person 1:	(+) or (-)	(+) or (-)	(+) or (-)
Person 2:	(+) or (-)	(+) or (-)	(+) or (-)
Person 3:	(+) or (-)	(+) or (-)	(+) or (-)
Person 4:	(+) or (-)	(+) or (-)	(+) or (-)
Person 5:	(+) or (-)	(+) or (-)	(+) or (-)

Step 4: Evaluate your results. Hopefully you chose your responses genuinely. If the majority of these people are producing positivity, that's amazing. Keep those people close! They will be an asset to you as you move towards your goals. If you're seeing a lot of negatives, it's time to reassess those around you. You don't need to excommunicate the bad eggs from your life, but you should find room for more people to serve you better. If you have negative influences around you, whether well intentioned or not, they're only going to hold you back. It's okay if Person Three moves to Person Six or Person Eight while you make some room for positive influences in your Circle of Success.

SUPER Action Step: Your Circle of Success is a fluid group of people that should be monitored from time to time. As you grow and evolve, your Circle should be doing the same. Your SUPER action is to revisit this POWER action every three months and constantly audit the people you keep closest to you.

Chapter 7

....

Fall in Love with the Process

Focus on the journey, not the destination.
Joy is found not in finishing an activity, but in doing it.

−Greg Anderson

A 39-year-old man stood at the podium, misty eyed. There were bulbs flashing, cameras recording, and a room full of reporters, friends, and family waiting to hear him speak. It had been 18 years since, as a rookie, he'd first stepped up to such a podium. This, as everyone had anticipated, was going to be his last.

In the time he spent in the NFL, he won the most MVP trophies (5), threw the most touchdowns (539), and accumulated the most passing yards (71,940) in history. These are only a few of the many records he holds. He capped his career with his second Super Bowl victory and rode off into the sunset as one of the best quarterbacks—if not *the* best—of all time. Peyton Manning was about to make it official; he had played his last game.

As he bid us farewell, he shared countless memories and moments that had made his career one of the most decorated of all time. It was the perfect ending to a near-perfect stint in the NFL.

From trainers to competitors, he spoke fondly of anyone who had crossed his path. He spoke of the low moments with humor, and the high moments with pride. He knew he'd had a good run. What stuck out to me, though, was how little he talked about his MVP awards or his Super Bowl championships. For someone who could have walked off of the field and immediately into the Hall of Fame, he could've spent all afternoon reviewing the highlights. Here's an excerpt where Manning talks about all the things he will miss about the game he loves:

When someone thoroughly exhausts an experience, they can't help but revere it. I revere football. I love the game. So you don't have to wonder if I'll miss it. Absolutely. Absolutely I will. Our children are small now, but as they grow up, we're going to teach them to enjoy the little things in life because one day they will look back and discover that those really were the big things. So here are the seemingly little things that when I look into my rearview mirror, have grown much bigger.

I'm going to miss a steak dinner at St. Elmo's in Indianapolis after a win. My battles with players named Lynch, Lewis, Thomas, Bruschi, Fletcher, Dawkins, Seau, Urlacher, Polamalu, Harrison, Woodson and Reed. And with coaches like Fisher, Ryan, Belichick, Kiffin, Phillips, Rivera, LeBeau, Crennel, Capers, Lewis, the late Jim Johnson, and so many more. I always felt like I was playing against that middle linebacker or that safety or that defensive coach.

I'll miss figuring out blitzes with Jeff Saturday. Reggie sitting on top of the bench next to me. Perfecting a fake handoff to Edgerrin James. I'll miss Demaryius Thomas telling me that he loved me and thanking me for coming to Denver after every touchdown I threw to him.

I'll miss putting in a play with Tom Moore and Adam Gase that ends in a touchdown on Sunday. On Fridays I'll miss picking out the game balls with my equipment guys. Talking football with the broadcast crews and, afterwards, I'll miss recapping the game with my dad. And checking to see if the Giants won and calling Eli as we're both on our team buses.

I'll miss that handshake with Tom Brady and I'll miss the plane rides after a big win with 53 teammates standing in the aisles, laughing and celebrating during the whole flight. I'll miss playing in front of so many great fans both at home and on the road. I'll even miss the Patriots fans in Foxborough, and they should miss me because they sure did get a lot of wins off of me.

Not *once* did he reference his two Super Bowl victories. No mention of the fact he is the only player in history to be honored as the Most Valuable Player in five seasons. No bragging about his slew of records. All Peyton Manning spoke about in his farewell speech was the journey. This man had more prizes, trophies, and accolades than anyone in the history of the game. But it was clear he loved the process of the game more than its prizes.

Fall in love with the process, not the prize. This is a concept I embed in my training philosophy. The truth is, the journey from where you are to the goal you want to achieve is a long one. The time you spend moving towards your goal will far outweigh the amount of time you spend enjoying it once you've actually accomplished it. If the majority of your time will be spent in the pursuit of your goal, you might as well learn to enjoy the rewarding process.

I have had tons of clients come to me with big goals. They want to lose 100 pounds, run a marathon, or drop a few dress sizes; I've seen it all. There's nothing wrong with goals. In fact, they're absolutely necessary. The problem I've seen, though, is some people get so obsessed with the end result, they miss out on the journey of getting themselves there. It's in this journey where the magic happens. It's within the process the prizes are earned. The process is what allows them to develop into the person worthy of achieving the lofty goal. I want my clients to reach every last one of their goals. But it's important they—and now you—understand that the commitment to the process is so much more important than the actual prize.

You know how Peyton Manning rose to be one of the best who ever played the game of football? It wasn't by obsessively focusing on winning a Super Bowl. It was by committing to—and subsequently enjoying—the details. He *enjoyed* late nights in the film room, studying opposing defenses. He *enjoyed* running through plays with his teammates until they got it just right. He *enjoyed* the competition. He *enjoyed* his failures because each one taught him something.

Other players may have begrudgingly suffered through those routine tasks, but Manning reveled in them. There was intrinsic value in perfecting the nuances of his game. He didn't show up day after day because he *had* to. He showed up to the film room, the practice field, and the weight room because he *wanted* to. It goes back to what we discussed about opportunity versus obligation in a previous chapter. Most people would see Manning's extra work, effort, and time as an obligation. He saw it as a grand opportunity. Another day to get better. Another day to fix a flaw. Another day to move himself closer to his goals. Yes, the Super Bowl victories and the MVP trophies may have been the goals. But what made the difference and, in retrospect, what Manning loved the most, were the small moments where he crafted his legacy. The early mornings and the late nights of hard work weren't only worth it, they were his favorite part.

There's a subtle difference between wanting to be a champion and wanting to be capable of a championship performance.

–Tom Bilyeu

Everyone is in love with the idea of success, but very few are willing to do the work necessary to achieve it. The trappings of perceived success trap all of us.

In your career, climbing the ladder to lead your company sounds amazing. Showing up at 5:00 a.m. every day to earn promotions doesn't. It's much easier to sneak in just as the workday starts and not make waves.

In your relationships, having a lifelong loving relationship with your spouse sounds incredible. Being vulnerable and trusting another human being with your love for the rest of your life is a bit less glamorous. It's scary. We can barely trust ourselves to take care of our well-being. Trusting another person can be a frightening proposition.

In your health, having a slim and beach-ready body sounds like a dream. Saying "no" to cookies or hitting the gym five times a week feels like a nightmare for some. Success takes sacrifice. It's much easier to be average, not having to push the boundaries of your comfort zone. Some people just aren't willing to do the work. Peyton Manning wasn't only willing; he loved it.

His records, his trophies, and his accolades were a direct result of the work he put in when no one was watching. If he had chosen to be satisfied with his skills as a rookie, his career wouldn't have been the same. I certainly wouldn't be writing about him in this book.

He unlocked a secret you can apply directly to any part of your life: **you are where you are in life because of *who* you are. If you're not where you want to be in life, it's because you're not who you need to be to get there.**

In order to do greater things, you have to become a greater person. Manning wanted to be a legend, so he developed legendary habits and skills. If you want more out of life, you have to grow to meet the challenge.

You have to shrink the space between your current self and your desired self. Who you are currently won't be able to do what's necessary to achieve your goals. You have to grow in order to reach something outside your current capacity.

The bridge between your current self and your desired self can be built with three main elements: decision, consistency, and resolve.

First, decide what you want. It could be a weight-loss goal, a relationship goal, or a professional goal; I don't care what it is. What's important is you make a firm decision on what it is and go after it. Write it down...in ink. You need to be all in when you decide because there is no turning back once you get moving.

Second, honor your decision and commitment with consistent action. There will be days when sleeping in will feel better than getting up and hitting the gym. Hell, to be honest, most days will feel that way.

If you've decided you're on a mission to lose weight, though, it doesn't matter. Get your ass out of bed and get to the gym. Destiny favors the committed. If you want to create serious change in your health, in your relationships, or in business, it requires daily, habitual, do-it-when-nobody's-looking work.

Finally, be resilient. You must have resolve. Whether you are an expert or an amateur, you will hit roadblocks. You will reach plateaus. You will want to quit.

Don't.

Find a different route. Find a way to transform the obstacles into allies. Use the frustration as fuel to keep moving. No matter what the problem, there is always a solution. Keep digging into the process until you find it.

These three elements will take you where you want to go. They will allow you to grow into the person you want to become.

You know what's funny, though? Peyton Manning could write a manual entitled *How to Become a Hall of Fame Quarterback*, but not everyone would cherish his advice. I could write an optimal nutrition and workout regimen for you, but you might not see the value in it.

Why? Because in both cases, the emphasis will be on the arduous long-term process. That's not sexy. No one wants to hear about all the minute details of success; they just like hearing about the culminating moment when it's realized.

The prizes of success *are* sexy: the slimmer, fitter body, the booming business, the nice house, the fancy car—the things everybody wants. Those rewards only come from a love affair with the dirty work. The small details of the process getting you there aren't optional; they are mandatory. They are absolutely necessary.

Fall in love with the journey. Fall in love with the early morning workouts. Fall in love with the great nutrition you use to fuel your body. Fall in love with the feeling of saying "no" to temptation. Get excited about the nuance of improved habits. Do the hard things until the hard things aren't hard anymore. This is the only way you will grow into the person capable of reaching your goal. There is no switch you can flip to take you from where you are now to the success you hope to achieve. The process will be a bumpy and winding path, but it will get you directly where you're trying to go. Embrace the journey.

There's no doubt embracing the small pieces of the process will get you to your goal. What's even more incredible is what you'll realize when you finally get there. Who you've become and what you've gone through will be more valuable to you than accomplishing what you've set out to do. Yes, being 100 pounds lighter will feel great. But what will feel better is your spouse saying, "You've changed through this process. You're happier. You're more alive. I like the new you, even without the weight loss."

You have to become a better version of yourself to create better results in your life. The transformation will emanate throughout all areas of your world, and you will look back on the arduous process and think, "Wow, that was amazing!" While making the choice to find more value in the journey, you'll ultimately find more value in yourself.

Testimonials from the Thrive Tribe

Meet Heather P.:

Over the years, I have wanted to be many things, but perfection was the thing I strived for the most. I've always felt I was a simple girl, there was nothing unique about me. I've never been extremely overweight, but I've never felt like I was the right size either. I have spent every moment from the age of twelve trying to find perfection, which really meant trying to be skinny. For some reason, I thought that if I was skinny, I'd have met my goal of being perfect. That is a lot of pressure to put on myself since I had only basic knowledge about health and nutrition. I tried all the fad diets. I tried many soup diets, I joined Jenny Craig twice. I joined Lindora and followed their plan. I even tried the cookie diet, twice.

Everything I tried worked! I lost weight, anywhere from 10–30 pounds, usually more than I realized I needed to lose. I would just start to feel better about my skinny self, then I'd go right back to my old ways of eating and quickly gain the weight back. It wasn't until I met Jay Nixon that I realized in order to be happy with the way I look on the outside, I had to fix me from the inside. I had no idea that was what Jay had been teaching me all along. Nineteen months ago, I walked into Jay's studio with plans to lose about 10 pounds. Instead, I have forever lost over 20 pounds, and I have gained the perfect idea of what healthy is. I am strong, I am fit, and I am awesome. I am healthy from within, and I've never felt better in my life.

My relationships with others, with food, and with myself have changed. I am still obsessed with being better, but I am happy with where I am and am loving how my personal changes have affected my family as well. They have a long way to go to get in the same mindset that Jay has put me in, but the way my husband and two young girls look at food and health has forever changed them, too. Thank you, Jay, for entering our lives.

Jay's Journal

It's who I am becoming through loving the process that matters. Today I will focus on mastering the process, and this will move me closer to the prize I desire, which is being my best self.

Your Journal

_____

_____

_____

_____

_____

Actions to Overcome the Overweight Mind

POWER Action Step: In the space provided, write down three health or fitness tasks you *hate* doing. I take no offense, I just want to see what parts of the process you currently dislike. On the right hand side, I want you to write down why you might be grateful for that task. You do not have to adore the action, but you can still find ways to understand why it might be a good thing for you. The examples on the left can be anything from working out in the morning, to eating less sugar, or going to bed earlier to get a good night's sleep. Do your best to find the good in each one. Write down why you're grateful for them and eventually you'll start falling hard for the process.

Things you dislike doing	Why you're grateful for the task
1) Preparing meals for the week	1) By preparing the meals proactively, I take the guesswork out of what I have to eat on a daily basis and set myself up for success.
2)	2)
3)	3)

SUPER Action Step: As you've read in this chapter, the process is where the magic happens. Use the table below to bridge the gap between your current self and your desired self by emphasizing the **process**. Use the example provided as a guide to create your own success map.

Current	Process for progress	Desired
Current Weight: 175	1) Exercise 4 days a week for 30 minutes 2) Stop eating dessert until I've reached my desired weight 3) Get 7–8 hours of sleep a night	Desired Weight: 140
Current _____	1) 2) 3)	Desired _____

Chapter 8

....

What You Do in the Dark

The difference between ordinary and extraordinary is that little extra.

–Jimmy Johnson

Peyton Manning's late nights in the film room behind closed doors created his legacy. Steve Jobs and Steve Wozniak spent endless hours holed up in Jobs's garage in the 1970s, planting the seeds of what has grown into the mammoth company known as Apple, Inc. Michael Phelps, the most decorated Olympian of all time, didn't earn his 23 gold medals in the spotlight of the Summer Olympics. It was the hard work he put in far away from the flashing lights and the medal ceremonies that created his rise to greatness. It's been said he swims six to eight hours a day, six days a week when in peak season. You don't see his training. You just see the triumphant celebration as they place another gold medal around his neck.

The point? Success isn't earned out in the open. It's earned in the moments behind closed doors when no one's watching. As you start down the path to a healthier lifestyle, this concept is paramount. Posting your progress pictures on Facebook or choosing the best filter for your healthy meal on Instagram isn't going to make a big difference in your long-term success. They might give you some positive feedback and make you feel good about what you're doing, but the likes and the comments aren't going to keep the weight off.

Having a public forum of people holding you accountable is great, but they won't be there when hunger strikes or you're feeling lethargic before a workout. What will you choose to eat? Will you choose to work out, or not? No one will know what you do. It's you versus you.

You get rewarded in public for what you do in private. Simple as that. A comment like, "Wow, you look GREAT" won't ever come your way unless you make GREAT decisions when no one's around. Your actions in private directly correlate to how good or bad your results are. Notice I said good OR bad. These moments of private action can work for or against you.

Let's highlight a moment we've all encountered before: the late-night snack. You wake up in the middle of the night and your stomach is just shouting at you. You feel you must appease it with something from the kitchen. Everyone's asleep. No one knows you're up. There are zero eyes on you. This moment is a microcosm of success or failure. Maybe you opt for a glass of cold water. Maybe you reach for something a little more filling, a little sweeter. Ice cream with a side of cookies. Why not? Because this private moment will spill into the public in due time.

Whether you choose the water or the ice cream topped with cookies, no one will ever know. You won't go on Facebook or Twitter and post, "Hey guys, I just opted to satisfy my late-night craving with a tall glass of water instead of a bowl of ice cream!" First, no one's up to see it. Second, most people won't really care about your moment of victory in the kitchen. They're too busy posting about politics or what their four-month-old kid likes to do (apparently it's not much more than eat, sleep, and poop). This moment is exclusively yours. No one will ever know what you choose. For now, anyway. Your choice will show itself over time.

Each time you choose the glass of water, you're making a small deposit into your "health bank." You're making a quality choice and, after enough deposits, the wealth you gain is the health you see. Each time you choose the ice cream, you're making a *withdrawal* from your "health bank." With each pint of ice cream you devour in the night, you're subtracting hard-earned gains and progress in your health and fitness. After enough withdrawals, you'll be left saying, "Where did my healthy body go?" It's a gradual process of improvement or deterioration. Consistency in either direction can make or break your healthy, fit body.

In truth, a glass of water is all you'll ever need to satisfy a late-night urge for consumption. Drink it down and let it settle. Your mind and body just needed a distraction in the middle of the night; the water will play that role just fine. If you choose to go for something more—a cookie, a banana, a bowl of ice cream—you are creating space for a new ritual. And the last thing you need is a late-night ritual involving sugary, calorie-heavy food.

> *A river cuts through rock, not because of its power,*
> *but because of its persistence.*
>
> –Jim Watkins

Like a river cutting through rock, your progress towards a healthy lifestyle and body will be decided by your consistent efforts. A river carves its way around and through rocks using time and persistence. Your body is the rock and your eating, exercise, and mindset habits are the river. It will take time, but with consistent effort and persistent application, you will carve out the health you desire.

It will take hundreds of good decisions, not just one or two. You can't expect a six-pack because you chose to start working out after 20 years of sedentary living. Ninety days of exercise won't cancel out the bad habits you've practiced for years. You need to give it time.

Similarly, one bad meal or cheat day isn't going to cancel out six months of hard work in the gym. Keep your "health bank" in mind here. The more deposits you make, the more you can afford a withdrawal here or there. If you've spent the last six months to a year eating well and exercising regularly, a weekend filled with greasy food and drinks won't cancel out all of your hard work. It will take some withdrawals away from the "health bank," but it won't decrease your balance to zero. It's a slippery slope, though. Don't let one weekend turn into a week, a month, or a year of indulgence. Your "health bank" will be empty before you know it, and you won't even realize all your credit is disappearing.

Think about your actual bank account. If you consistently put money in without taking much out, your wealth will grow over time. If you keep making withdrawals and only make a deposit here and there, your wealth will remain stagnant. Those repeated deposits day after day, week after week, will eventually pay huge dividends. Every time you make a withdrawal, you're threatening the progress of your wealth accumulation. And that's if you're starting from zero. If you're in debt, your wealth can't grow until you've paid back the money you owe. Once you get squared away, you can begin to build and accumulate wealth over time.

Your "health bank" operates in the same fashion. Make deposits consistently and you'll see progress. Make enough withdrawals and you'll see your health deteriorate. And the debt? That's when you've been ignoring your health, or treating it so badly you have to put in work to get back to square one.

Some of my clients get frustrated when they don't see progress fast enough. They've come to me 75 pounds overweight and expect to lose it all in a few months. They've been accumulating debt in their "health bank" for so long they have to "get back to even" before they can accumulate the wealth of health they deserve.

Consistency is key. To harness the power of a healthy body, you need to make quality choices every single day when no one is watching. Making those deposits into your "health bank" will produce rewards over time.

Remember: **you get rewarded in public for what you do in private.**

Be persistent in private. Know your continued efforts will create amazing changes in your life if you're willing to see the process through. What you do in the dark will be shown in the light. Not tomorrow or the next day, but give it time. Be the river that cuts through rock.

Testimonials from the Thrive Tribe

Meet Anisa S.:

People often asked how I lost 56 pounds. My response usually goes, "With hard work, perseverance, determination, and consistency." I always refer back to Jay Nixon and how his program has changed my life in many ways.

The person I am today is not the person I was a year ago. I have had a complete transformation, not just physically, but personally as well. When I walked into the studio on the first day, I was overweight, dealing with PCOS, irregular cycles, borderline diabetic, depressed, mourning the loss of a child, going through a divorce, and completing my Master's degree. I was never putting myself first. I accommodated people to appease them. It was starting to take a toll on me. I was becoming a person I did not like at all. At 33 years old I felt completely lost in life. I had no idea where my journey was going to take me. I thought the first thing to help myself was to get healthy.

The first day I wanted to throw up and couldn't even complete a lap. Yes, I had "worked out" before, but never at the intensity of my first day with Jay. I can honestly say I hated the process at first. The first few months into the program, I just coasted. I was still very insecure about myself and doubted myself daily. I would make excuses as to why I didn't want to work out or why the eating was too hard. After talking to Jay about some personal issues and how to deal with problems in my life, I was better able to handle them with ease and a sense of calmness. I knew I needed to put myself first in life before I could help others.

The first step was to zone in on my fitness and nutrition. I was working out one day and it just clicked. I wanted to be happy and I knew my "WHY." After that, I fell in love with the process. I woke every morning at 4:30 a.m. and worked out. I gave one hundred percent of myself to get better every day. Before I could realize what was happening, I was running faster, picking up heavier weights, and pushing myself. Jay always says, "You must fall in love with the process to reap the benefits." Jay has saved my life and I am thankful for him every day. He is not just a personal trainer, I am blessed to call him my friend. The person I am today is happy, healthy, fit, confident, and strong. I deal with life situations differently and it has made relationships better in my life. I went from 175 pounds to 119 pounds. I look at myself and I don't recognize the person I once was. I love myself now and that is the greatest gift I could have ever given myself. If I had the opportunity to go back and talk to the "pre-transformation" me, I would tell her, "You are worth it, you can do it, and you are amazing." The accomplishments and pride of getting fit is worth the discomfort you will experience at first. I wake up cheerful, confident, and ready to conquer the day because of the guidance of Jay, who I like to call my life coach.

Jay's Journal

It's not one big thing that makes you successful. I know my success is dependent on consistently doing the little things day in and day out. Today I will master the little things.

Your Journal

_____

_____

_____

_____

_____

Actions to Overcome the Overweight Mind

POWER Action Step: I want you to keep a running log of the small actions you take when no one's looking. Find an app on your phone or keep a small journal on you at all times. Every time you opt for vegetables over fries at a restaurant, make note of it. Every time you go for a run when you didn't really feel like it, write it down. By keeping this continuous log, you are building *evidence* that proves you CAN make the tough decisions when no one's watching. This evidence will propel you forward with the confidence that you can and will stay on track towards your goals. Get that app up and running today!

SUPER Action Step: Right now, chances are you have some guilty pleasures you enjoy away from the public eye when you're stressed, depressed, or emotional. Use the space below to record and plan the behavioral shift that will empower the actions you take in private.

Example of Current Behavior: You overindulge in comfort foods at the end of a high-stress work day.

Shift to New Behavior: To diffuse the stress of your work day, you should go for a hike or do a quick 30-minute workout. This change in your physical state will make you feel SO much better than the food that was supposed to bring you "comfort."

Current Behavior:

Shift to New Behavior:

Chapter 9

Fueling Your Body versus Failing Your Body

Every time you eat or drink, you are either feeding disease or fighting it.
−Heather Morgan

A man stands alone in a kitchen. He looks up at the camera and says, "Is there anyone out there who still isn't clear about what doing drugs does? Okay, last time." He walks over to the stove, picks up an egg, and continues, "This is your brain." He points to a frying pan on a burner. "This is drugs." He cracks the egg and lets it begin to sizzle on the hot pan, egg whites and yolk bubbling from the heat. "This is your brain on drugs. Any questions?"

This iconic commercial from the 1980s was created to showcase the damage drugs can do to your brain. The analogy may not have been spot on, but the imagery was enough to make people think twice before taking a harmful substance. By now, everyone understands the risks and dangers of taking drugs like cocaine or heroin. With Google at our fingertips everywhere we go, it's not difficult to figure out why it wouldn't be a good idea. These drugs are damaging and addictive, creating a vicious cycle of dependency leading to destruction.

What if I told you your brain reacts to heroin and cocaine in the same way it reacts to some of the foods you eat on a daily basis? This isn't a scare tactic. I have science in my corner. Several studies over the past decade indicate the brain's reaction to sugar eerily mimics its response to heroin or cocaine. I'll say it again—maybe it will sink in—your brain reacts to sugar like it does to cocaine and heroin.

If you want to dive into all the science behind the scenes, you can find the research articles in the reference section at the back of the book.

The comparison between your brain's reaction to drugs and sugar is twofold. First, there are similarities in the consumption of the two. Second, there is a link between the addiction cycles formed from both.

Let's start with the physical consumption of a drug like heroin or cocaine in comparison to the intake of sugar. Dopamine is a substance in your brain that is associated with pleasure, therefore an increase of it means an increase in pleasure. A recent study shows that eating something high in sugar and taking a hit of cocaine result in similar increases of dopamine in your brain. This would explain the high of taking drugs and the feeling of temporary ecstasy often paired with the experience. It's the rush of pleasure that accompanies the consumption of a sugary, sweet donut or cookie. You know the audible sigh of bliss you exhale when you bite into a brownie or a piece of cake? That's the dopamine increase in your brain telling you, "This is SO good!"

The increase in dopamine and the feeling of pleasure is one thing, but it's not the worst part about the similarities.

What is amazing about the human body is its constant efforts to normalize your levels of pain and pleasure. It never wants you to experience too much of either extreme because it could spell disaster for your health. Think about when you jump into a pool or the ocean and the chill of the water catches you off guard. When you first enter, it feels frigid. But, over time, your body gets *used to it*. The water didn't get warmer, your body just adjusted so you didn't feel too cold while you splashed around.

Your body does the same thing with the consumption of drugs or sugary sweets. Over time, it will get used to the increases of dopamine and other pleasure-related substances and begin to anticipate the spike. When your brain senses the trigger of your drug or sugar habit loop, it will decrease the substances related to pleasure to offset the anticipated increase. Meaning, as soon as you see the box of donuts or Girl Scout cookies, your brain will decrease those substances it expects will soon increase. The same thing happens when a drug addict sees their pipe or smells the scent of their drug of choice.

This can do one of two things. If a drug or donut is consumed, it doesn't produce the pleasure it once did. Then what happens? Well, you naturally compensate for the unimpressive joy you received from the indulgence and consume more. Focusing on your food intake here, that means you'll need more food—specifically unhealthy, processed food—to make your brain happy. While attempting to appease the brain and hit the previous high you had, you'll consume more calories and more processed food. Your mind is leading you right into obesity without you even knowing it!

Now, let's take a look at what happens if you resist the urge to take the drugs or to consume the sugar-laced food after previously indulging. As stated before, your body will still anticipate the consumption based on previous experience. When it anticipates the rush of dopamine and other pleasure-related substances, it will proactively *decrease* the levels in your body to offset the impending spike. But, you reject the urge to have the donut. Your body has lowered its blood sugar and pleasure substances in anticipation of your habit, but now you've left it hanging. This will result in decreased energy in the effort to say no. Plus, you're hungrier than ever. It will be much harder to resist the cravings because you've created a gap between what your brain thinks is normal and your current state. Since the brain's reaction to sugar-laced foods is so similar to that of taking drugs, resisting the urge to binge eat has become as hard as quitting cocaine or heroin cold turkey.

As I said before, everyone is aware of the addictive and destructive cycles drugs can create. What most don't understand—and by now I hope you do—is how your consumption of foods laced with sugar can create an equally damaging cycle. Even with this scientific evidence, a great many people avoid coming to terms with the severity of the sugar rush.

"One donut won't hurt."

"I can have a cookie every now and again."

Can a crack addict have a hit every once in a while? Should someone trying to eliminate a heroin addiction take some in moderation? OF COURSE NOT. We, as a culture, need to see sugar addiction in the same light. If you have a problem consuming cookies at night, get them out of your house. If you can't hold back from digging into a pint of ice cream, remove it from your freezer. Out of sight, out of mind. Keeping sugary treats around won't allow you to step away from your bad habit. Someone with a drug addiction can't have their drug of choice close by if they're trying to quit. Do the same for yourself if there is a particular food or snack you are having trouble kicking.

With the addictive cycle sugar can create, a constant part of the habit loop is food consumption. Your brain gets tricked into needing and wanting more, so you're left on autopilot, unconsciously shoveling in more calories to satisfy your brain chemicals. Keep this in mind when you reach for the next handful of Oreos or Hershey Kisses. You are opening a cycle leading you down a road of subconscious consumption.

> *The food you eat can either be the safest and most powerful*
> *form of medicine, or the slowest form of poison.*
> –Ann Wigmore

Let this information empower you. Take it and use it as a weapon against the tyranny of big name companies spending millions of dollars on advertisements for their over-processed, sugar-laced food.

There's a negative correlation between dollars spent in advertising and the quality of nutrition in a given product. In other words, the more a company spends shoving a product down your throat, the worse its nutritional value.

Have you ever seen a Super Bowl commercial for broccoli? My point exactly. Stick with broccoli and avoid the pizza. Choose fresh greens over salty chips. Go with cauliflower and steer clear of the candy aisle.

Your food choice will make or break your health. This isn't just about looking good, it's about living a long, vibrant life. Type 2 diabetes, the leading type of diabetes in the United States, has links to obesity. If you can control your weight and fend off obesity—and in turn type 2 diabetes—by choosing quality nutrition, why wouldn't you?

There are also studies speculating that Alzheimer's disease could be a third type of diabetes. Diabetes is a direct or indirect cause of death for over 200,000 Americans each year. By controlling your food choices, you can prevent becoming overweight and obese—and you might be able to avoid Alzheimer's as well. While the jury is still out on the last one, why take a chance?

Connect the dots and understand how important it is to put quality food in your body. Your food is your fuel. You can either put some high-performance fuel in your engine, or you can opt for toxic sludge.

I do what I do not only to get my clients in shape but also because I want them to live long, healthy lives. Nutrition is SO important on so many levels. Nutrition intake is a form of mechanics, which may seem off-theme for this book. But the research in this chapter shows you just how much nutrition can impact your mind. Choosing processed food affects your brain and causes subconscious, repeated consumption. Overconsumption and cyclical indulging can slowly but surely lead you to obesity. Being overweight or obese enhances the possibility of diabetes. It all starts with the food you are *choosing* to put in your body.

Start eating with intention and get off autopilot.

Stop *failing* your body and start *fueling* your body.

Testimonials from the Thrive Tribe

Meet Annie M:

I'm thankful for Jay Nixon—WOW! I know I am a newbie, but the impact you have had on me, my journey, and my family is immeasurable. In so many ways you have changed my outlook on life, work, and relationships. I work harder, eat better, love bigger, and enjoy life 100% more.

You have impacted the health and wellness of my husband as well as my own. He has lost over 30 pounds and is no longer taking blood pressure medicine. He will even be running a 1/2 marathon soon! My kids (five and seven) are learning about health and how important it is. They're learning about what sugar can do to your brain and your body. Giving them this awareness at such a young age is a blessing. On days when I'm not in the studio with the Thrive Tribe, my children come to the garage and do their own version of jumping jacks and burpees.

Stepping on the scale used to scare me; now I don't care because I know if my eating is on point and I work out hard every day, I will CRUSH my MUSTS! So, thank you for creating this tribe of badass, beautiful people. Thanks for caring so much about our success. I am so lucky to be a part of this tribe!

Jay's Journal

My body and brain combine to form a perfect machine, and I must nourish the machine with great food and great ideas. Treating my body like a precious gift will allow me to perform at my maximum potential. I know the food I eat affects the way my body feels and how my brain functions. I will only eat foods that give me energy and allow me to perform and think at my highest level.

Your Journal

_____

_____

_____

_____

_____

_____

Actions to Overcome the Overweight Mind

POWER Action Step: This task is simple: list three foods you know are like a drug to you on the left. These three foods GOTTA GO. Get them out of your sight path and away from your nostrils. On the right-hand side, write three foods of quality nutrition you will acquire to fill the void in your home. Once you've completed your list, take ACTION and make the transition to a healthier kitchen!

Foods That I'm Addicted To (Bad Options)	Better Choices (Healthy Options)
1) Chocolate Chip Cookie	1) A square of 90% Dark Chocolate
2)	2)
3)	3)

SUPER Action Step: List your meals for the day and then use the rating scale provided to assess how those food decisions made you feel. The purpose of this exercise is to make you more mindful of the things you eat and then connect them to your emotions. Mindful consumption is a catalyst to *fueling* your body properly.

Meal	How You Feel 1-Stuffed, Gassy, Lethargic, Bloated, Need a Nap 2-Full, Low Energy, Sluggish 3-Content, Average Energy 4-Satisfied, High Energy, Fueled
Breakfast: Oatmeal with blueberries, coffee with cream and sugar	2
Lunch: Chopped salad, no cheese, sparkling water with lemon	4
Dinner: Pizza and chicken wings, two beers	1

Meal	How You Feel 1-Stuffed, Gassy, Lethargic, Bloated, Need a Nap 2-Full, Low Energy, Sluggish 3-Content, Average Energy 4-Satisfied, High Energy, Fueled
Breakfast:	
Lunch:	
Dinner:	

Chapter 10

....

There is No Finish Line

Without continual growth and progress, such words as improvement,
achievement, and success have no meaning.

–Benjamin Franklin

On August 1, 2015, two opponents met in the middle of the ring in Rio de Janeiro. The referee was going to the winner. One person stepped to the middle with swagger; the other was dejected, knowing she'd squandered the chance to dethrone the queen of the UFC, Ronda Rousey. The ref raised Rousey's hand to announce her victory, which most had seen as inevitable from the start.

Rousey had never lost as a professional mixed martial arts fighter. In this particular fight, she knocked out her opponent, Bethe Correia, in 34 seconds. More impressively, this particular victory took longer to claim than in her previous two fights *combined*. Her previous two matches lasted a punctual 14 and 16 seconds respectively. As she stood next to Correia, securing yet another win, Rousey was on top of the UFC world. She seemed unstoppable. She seemed unbeatable. She seemed inhuman.

But, just a few months later, one kick reestablished her mortality.

As she made a name for herself in the UFC, Ronda Rousey's star began to rise in the public eye. She did plenty of late-night talk shows and interviews and even landed a role in the action movie *Furious 7*. With all of the extracurricular activities, you have to wonder the effect on her training. The amount of work she put in to get to the top of the mountain must've been massive. Something had to take a back seat to her outside-the-ring activities.

Well, on November 14th, roughly three months after she knocked out her opponent in just 34 seconds, she found herself on the other end of the foot. Holly Holm, a prohibitive underdog, knocked Rousey out with a swift kick to the head. It was a devastating blow to Rousey's physical body and to her ego. She hasn't won a fight since; who knows if she ever will.

So, what happened? Was she not as good as we all thought? Was she overrated? No, not at all. She was taking care of her competition with ease up until that point.

It's simple, really: she let her guard down. Sure, she physically let it down, which opened a window of opportunity for Holm's infamous kick. More importantly, though, Rousey eased up in her preparation. She eased up in her training. She let the edge of her killer instinct grow dull. Her mastery of the craft became her greatest enemy.

Once Rousey reached a certain level of dominance, she stopped putting in the work that had gotten her there. She assumed she could just continue to walk in and beat every woman she faced in less than a minute. By allowing the spotlight to distract her from her characteristic hard work, she left herself open for a downfall.

Ronda Rousey isn't the first person to meet this fate. There are plenty of examples of people who have fallen from greatness in shocking fashion. No matter who you are, or what you're trying to accomplish…

...in order to be successful, and to REMAIN successful, you must continue to seek growth and be willing to learn more.

If you let up because you think you've "made it," you're going to be in trouble. Once you stop putting in the work that produced your success, you can't expect success to keep coming your way. I understand most of my readers aren't looking to become professional athletes or UFC fighters, but this cautionary tale can be applied to any goal you have.

In the realm of health and fitness, this model of continual growth is a *must*. The reason I don't let my clients use the word "diet" is because of the time constraints usually paired with it. If you come to me and say, "I want to diet to look good for my wedding," we're going to have some problems. Look, I am 100% in favor of quality nutrition, but the wedding (or vacation, or high school reunion) you're preparing for promotes a subconscious deadline. As soon as the day comes, you'll throw your habits out the window and start destroying any progress you've made. The hard work that produced your results will cease and you will see your progress vanish.

Living a healthy lifestyle has no deadline. There is no finish line to cross, making it okay to stop exercising or eating well. Healthy living is a continuous process that is never complete. That's why I laugh at all the 60-day and 90-day workout plans guaranteeing a healthy new you. They will most likely produce a fitter version of you, but there's no way your *health* will be forever changed in that timeframe.

Your health is something you should be working on from now until the day you die. The work shouldn't end after just three months.

I apply the approach of continual improvement to every aspect of my life. With my business and in building the Thrive Tribe, I'm always looking for ways to improve. I don't just come up with one workout or nutrition plan and then go through the motions. I'm constantly researching, upgrading, and reinventing my program so it is always optimal for my clients. I've had some clients for *years*, and I would be doing them an absolute disservice if I were to bring them the same product and the same energy every year. In order to thrive as much as my Tribe's title would suggest, I'm in a constant state of progress.

Outside of my business, I have invested thousands of dollars in mastermind groups, personal development conferences, and personal coaching. I am constantly looking to better myself through these experiences so it will cause a ripple effect of excellence throughout my life.

I always tell my clients, "Never trust a coach who doesn't have a coach." If I don't have someone I consult for feedback and advice, how can I ask you to? If I'm not being mentored by someone else, I am allowing my knowledge and abilities to stagnate. The more stagnant I am, the less I can do for you. My clients will always get the best out of me because I'm always seeking ways to get better.

Look at the best athletes in the world. All of them have coaches they respect. All of them seek advice from mentors either in-house or through private training. The reason they are at the top level is because they sought the help they needed to fine tune the nuances of their individual games.

Some may think LeBron James doesn't need a coach. He does, but for different reasons than his peers. While his teammates are working on their shooting or their dribbling, LeBron is working with someone to improve his mental edge or situational tactics. He's farther down the rabbit hole of basketball training, but he still needs guidance.

Tom Brady is an incredible quarterback, but his dominance has been aided by having an all-time great coach on the sidelines in Bill Belichick. Brady would still be great without the coach, but having Belichick to help with the intricate details of the game helped immensely.

Coaches, mentors—anyone who holds you accountable as you strive for success—are essential. One thing you want to avoid, though, is recruiting a friend, family member, or spouse to be responsible for your continued growth and expansion. Your family and friends should be your cheerleaders, not your coach. Obviously, on a sports team, a coach and a cheerleader play very different roles, and for good reason. A coach's job is to get in your ear and give you objective advice on how to improve. A cheerleader's job is to support you and to cheer for you. Your friends and family members are too close to you to be objective. They'll hold back when asked to keep you accountable. They'll ease up when something needs critiquing. Keep your coaches and cheerleaders separate. You need someone in your corner who will build you up, not just cheer for you.

> *The more you know, the more you know you don't know.*
> —Aristotle

As you begin (and then continue) your journey to a healthier body and a healthier you, keep Aristotle's quotation in mind. The farther you get into the process, the more there is to learn.

Take nutrition as a small example: At first you may master the relationship of calories in versus calories out. Then, you will learn to understand macronutrients and how to balance them in your meals. Once you figure that out, you'll learn more about the power of micronutrients and all they can do for your health. The farther down the road you get, the more experience and more knowledge you'll have. But you'll also see how much more there is to learn.

A deep exploration of nutrition, fitness, and personal development can seem overwhelming. With so many avenues to explore, it's even more important to have a coach or a mentor to light the way. By investing in someone who's been there before, you can save yourself time, trial, and error. Working with a coach is the most-efficient avenue to accelerate and continue your growth.

I continue to have coaches and mastermind groups around me. They keep me focused on my goals and help me avoid mistakes I would've made on my own.

If you're looking for a coach or a tribe to rally around you, don't hesitate to contact me at www.JOINTHETHRIVETRIBE.com. The Thrive Tribe is family to me and it will be the same for you. We are a group of committed people working towards becoming our best selves every single day. The community we've created is special and will give you insight into the best health and fitness information. In addition, we will provide support as you move towards your goals.

I'd be honored to stand with you as you look to better yourself. Even if you choose someone else, find yourself a coach or mentor. We do so much more than get you to your goal; we help you with the next one...and the next...and the next.

You may come to me hoping to lose 30 pounds. I can absolutely help you, but I want to do so much more. Those 30 pounds will be nothing in comparison to the lifestyle changes I can help you create. I want you to relish in your accomplishments AND the person you've become in the process. I want you to create future goals, too, whether they involve keeping the 30 pounds off, working on muscle tone, or helping to find your passion in life.

My job, and the job of any coach, is to help you raise your standard of living. I'm going to help you eat better, exercise more, and live a more fulfilling life. I'm going to hold you accountable to your goals and keep you on track to reach them.

What's beautiful about having a coach, a mentor, or a fine-tuned Circle of Success is that everyone's success is tied together. I've seen it through my own personal experience. My coaches and mentors love it when I succeed because it means they've done their jobs. If I help you become successful with your goals, I share your level of success. Helping people live their best life possible is my "why." It's what gets me up in the morning, fired up and ready to start the day.

Seek people like me who will stand in your corner and help push you to achieve your goals. Keep looking to better yourself. Keep growing. The day you find yourself in a state of stagnation is the day you begin to regress. To keep your trajectory pointed upward, recruit people to build you up to the person you want to be.

The "do-it-yourself" model of progress can only get you so far. Investment in people and activities can and will accelerate your expansion.

In this world, you're either growing or you're dying,
so get in motion and grow.

–Lou Holtz

Your goals are not finish lines; they are checkpoints. Losing 30 pounds isn't the end of the road—it's just a beginning. More goals will follow and more growth will be needed. Your new goal might be a performance goal like running a half marathon or competing in a CrossFit competition. It could be to gain more muscle tone or to lose more weight. Celebrate each checkpoint, but know you're never done. There is no finish line.

Ronda Rousey thought her work was done, but Holly Holm showed her there's always more work to do. Don't make the "Rousey" mistake. Seek continual growth with the help of an experienced mentor who can accelerate and multiply it. You are more than worth the investment.

Testimonials from the Thrive Tribe

Meet Cherylynn C.:

I won two free sessions with Jay, December of 2015. I went to my first workout with him. I thought I was going to die. I think I did actually. That was the hardest workout I had ever done in my life. I didn't go back for the second workout. Maybe it showed how much I was out of shape. Maybe it showed how I needed change. I wasn't ready for Jay.

In May of 2016, a friend of mine approached me about joining Jay's program. I was not sure I wanted to, of course. Not sure I could fit it into my schedule of work, three kids, and their extracurricular activities. Not sure if I could afford it. Not sure. With much reluctance and encouragement, I joined. I laugh about how I started with Jay, the day I went in for my measurements. I knew what to do. I knew what to eat. I knew. He was very patient, listening to what I was saying. Asking me what my goal was. I just wanted to lose weight, 20–30 pounds.

Every week I died during his workouts. Eventually I started feeling stronger. My clothes started to fit looser. I felt different, stronger, and happier. The workouts are only a part of the process. I learned how to eat. I learned about what food really was, what was better for me and what wasn't. I've learned to "stay in my lane" and to know when I need to reach out for help. I get support and encouragement from Jay and his Facebook group. Jay is so knowledgeable and he helps guide us into making better choices by educating. He doesn't say things without explanation. He backs up his information.

I rely on the support of our group. My days aren't perfect, but they're better than they were before Jay. It's important to have like-minded people in your life to keep you moving in the same direction you want to go. They keep the positive vibes going, they give you support when you're feeling down. So what started as a weight-loss program has turned into a lifestyle program. I've lost 30 pounds, but gained so much knowledge. My belly no longer gets in the way of my seat belt. I've gotten rid of my pre-pregnancy fat clothes.

I'm learning I can be, do, and have anything I want. I'm forever thankful for Jay and what he does to help people. He is an amazing and selfless nutritionist, coach, and friend!

Jay's Journal

Progress equals success. Today I will surround myself with positive people, positive conversation, and positive actions and this positive proximity will allow me to move forward on my journey to greatness.

Your Journal

_____

_____

_____

_____

_____

_____

_____

Actions to Overcome the Overweight Mind

POWER Action Step: Identify one area of your life where you need mentorship. I know this book is health- and fitness-oriented, but I want you to level up your entire life, so examine your entire spectrum. You might need a personal trainer, a relationship counselor, or a nutritionist; it doesn't matter. Write down what you need, then write the target date by which you will invest in solving your need.

Type of Coach/Mentor_____ Deadline to hire

_____

SUPER Action Step: In the space provided, write down an area of your life where you've become stagnant. Look, this is your book, so be honest with what you write down. No one's asking you to say it out loud in front of a crowd. It could be health, fitness, relationships, or your career; just write down an area you've neglected for a while.

Area of Stagnation

Now write down what you could do to work on this area of your life. If it's your relationships, write down actions you can take to better them. If it's your career, write down actions you can take to show up in a bigger way. If it's your health, write down actions you need to focus on to improve the stagnant nature of it. The key is *action*.

Chapter 11

Your Upgrade Is Now Available

Change is inevitable. Growth is optional.

–John Maxwell

Your phone lights up.

"New update available. Download now."

Without hesitation, you opt to update. With a simple click of a button, your phone has turned into a newer, more efficient machine. It's fine-tuned any bugs in its system, gotten rid of anything that was slowing it down, and has developed new features that will keep it performing at a high level in today's ever-changing world.

With your newer, better phone you decide to start researching new cars on the Internet. It's time to change your ride. You're ready for something fresh and vibrant, new car smell included. You find a car you like at a local dealer, set up an appointment, and head over to negotiate a deal. In just a few hours, you drive away with your brand new car, paired with a smile from ear to ear.

On the way home, you spot a sign on a quiet street that reads, "Open House." You and your spouse have been thinking about upgrading your living quarters for a while, so you stop in and have a look. It's the perfect size. The master bedroom is spectacular. The open floor plan is incredible. You both love the place and put in an offer before you leave.

What a day! You updated your phone to the latest and greatest features, bought a new car, and made an offer on your dream home.

As you wind down from such an amazing day, you catch a glimpse of yourself in the mirror. You see a little flab where there wasn't any a few months ago. You think to yourself:

"Maybe I shouldn't have had that third piece of cake. I should probably get back in the gym."

Then you keep walking, not giving much thought to your humbling encounter with your reflection. After upgrading everything in your life in one day, you don't give any consideration to upgrading *yourself*. You don't think twice when improving your cell phone, your car, your house, or any other aspect of your life. But when it comes time to hit the "upgrade" button on yourself, you hesitate. You *do* think twice, then a third and a fourth time. Eventually, you decide the comfort zone you occupy is cozy. Let's not push it, life is pretty good.

The following excerpt from Steven Kotler and Jamie Wheal's book, *Stealing Fire*, speaks directly to our culture's resistance to upgrade:

> *One in three Americans, for example, is obese or morbidly obese, even though we have access to better nutrition at lower cost than any time in history. Eight out of ten of us are engaged or actively disengaged at work, despite the HR circus of incentive plans, team-building off-sites, and casual Fridays. Big-box health clubs oversell member-ships by 400% in the certain knowledge that, other than the first two weeks in January and a brief blip before spring break, fewer than one*

in ten members will ever show up. And when a Harvard Medical School study confronted patients with lifestyle-related diseases that would kill them if they didn't alter their behavior (type 2 diabetes, smoking, atherosclerosis, etc.), 87 percent couldn't avoid this sentence. Turns out, we'd rather die than change.

The problem with the passive logic shown in Kotler and Wheal's passage and in our culture at large is that all of the other upgrades aren't nearly as useful as the ones you can make to yourself. Upgrading your phone or driving away in a brand new car may bring a temporary rush of happiness, but it won't last long. Wait until the next best thing comes out and watch how you'll be itching to upgrade once again.

Upgrading yourself, however, is a process promising continual fulfillment. With each goal you set and accomplish, with each milestone you reach, you are providing meaningful feedback to yourself that screams, "I can do it! I am worthy! Life is good!" If you settle on the current version of yourself, you won't get the same results. If you don't continually upgrade and work on your body and mind, there's no feedback. There's no information proving or disproving you're worthy of what you have or what you want.

Think about the current phone you have or the car you currently drive. These two objects of your affection are probably the best examples because of how quickly value depreciates. Whether it be the model or software of your phone, how quickly do the features become obsolete? Manufacturers come out with a new smart phone every year or so, each one debuting startling new features. First came emoji's, then Siri, and now if you text someone "Happy Birthday," your phone cues up some fireworks to play in the background of your birthday message. That's just the cute stuff.

Each time Apple debuts its newest creation, there are tons of practical advantages to buying the new one and discarding the old one. It could be the camera, battery life, or a multitude of other features, but we trust developers are pushing the envelope with each new release. So, without fail, we wait in line to pay hundreds of dollars for the upgrade. Having an iPhone 5 when the iPhone 7 just came out can be social suicide in some circles.

Then there's the brand new car you've been eyeing. It's a thing of beauty, isn't it? You deserve such a nice ride. It has all of the bells and whistles…for now. As soon as you drive it off the lot, you've lost so much monetary value it's as if the dealership just stole thousands from you. Give it a few years and all of the state-of-the-art automotive features will become a thing of the past as the next wave of brand new cars hits the market. So again, without fail, you decide to upgrade.

With cars and phones, you trade-in, trade-up, and upgrade as much as possible. You don't want to be stuck in the past with an outdated product. But why is it so easy to upgrade things but not yourself?

We live in a world of instant gratification. You can very easily update or upgrade your phone, your car, and potentially your home in one day's time. Self-help gurus, fitness professionals, and other marketers will try to sell you a quick-fix personal upgrade knowing "fast and furious" sells in our society.

Here's your wake-up call. Lasting mental and physical health represent a continuous process—there is no finish line. Good health is not something you achieve after reading one book or completing one 60-day weight-loss program. Upgrading the way you think, the way you eat, and other habitual routines takes time—a lot of time.

The never-ending timeline of personal growth runs contrary to the world around us. That's why we all hesitate to hit the "upgrade" button for ourselves. We're used to having what we want within minutes or hours. We make a choice—change occurs. It just simply doesn't work like that when it comes to becoming your best self.

Upgrading to the best version of YOU requires investment on a *continuing daily* basis.

Move your body every day. It could be a rigorous form of exercise or a leisurely walk around your neighborhood, but find a way to raise your heart rate. Eat quality foods every single day. Don't eat healthy during the work week and then trash it all on the weekend.

Read a quality personal development book every day. Just ten pages a day is fine. If you make this a daily habit, you'll read about 300 pages a month, which is about one book. The reason I find reading so vital to my own personal growth is because it continually broadens my perspective of my psychology and mindset. The more books you read, the more insight you can download into your brain. If you're not a fan of reading words on a page, you can always listen to audiobooks or podcasts. Anything engaging your mind and pushing the boundaries of what you think you know will prove beneficial.

Things like cellphones, cars, and houses are in constant need of upgrade for good reason. As the customer, we demand more of the companies who sell to us. We want the fastest, coolest, most-efficient versions of whatever we buy. On the flip side, the companies we frequent continue to raise the bar of "the possible." They are always one step ahead of us, creating amazing products we didn't even think we needed.

You have more computing power in your hand than the president of the United States had at his disposal just a few decades ago. Your car will soon be driving itself. Your home's security, lighting, and heat can all be controlled from the super-powered cellphone in your hand. Companies and consumers work to create a melting pot of forward momentum, leading the world around us towards consistent improvement.

Pay attention here—you are *both* the company and the consumer. You are the one creating the product and the one enjoying the results. Push the boundaries of your comfort zone and keep looking to update your current settings. If you don't, no one else will. The only person who can create the atmosphere of constant physical/mental upgrades is you. You need to *demand* a better version of yourself, and you *supply* it through hard work and perseverance.

Don't allow your body to become the equivalent of a 1995 Ford Explorer or a "bag phone." Don't accept personal obsolescence. Accept, embrace, and pursue personal change.

Upgrade your mindset

Understand you are capable of making lasting health changes in your life. You may hit roadblocks or reach plateaus but don't let negative thoughts take control. Use your mind to serve you, not to hold you captive as you strive for your goals.

Increase your "why." Dig deep and understand exactly why you want to make big changes in your health and fitness. Don't settle for "I want to lose 20 pounds." Push to find the "I want to live longer than my dad who died young of heart disease" or "I want to be a positive role model for my children." Upgrade your "why" so you have a crystal clear vision of what brings you to the gym each morning and what keeps you away from the fridge late at night.

Upgrade your habits

Make sure your habits are serving you in every way possible. Create habits that promote health and vitality and change those threatening to derail your progress. You have the power to change your habits, you just need to put in the effort.

Binge on books, not on Netflix. Silence stress with exercise, not with ice cream. Build your life up with the best habits you can. Your habits are a subconscious robot controlling most of your daily function. Since you can program a robot to help you instead of hurt you, take advantage.

Upgrade your emotional awareness

Recognize when you are eating because you're sad, not hungry. Identify the differences and make note of them. Experiment with different triggers and solutions so you can control your emotional eating. Get in touch with your "easy buttons." Become more aware of when you are using food to fill a void or a need in your life. Keep a journal tracking your emotions in relation to your meals. This will help increase the awareness you need to make any changes.

Upgrade your beliefs, thoughts, and vocabulary

It all starts with your beliefs and builds from there. If your beliefs are out of date, it's time to change them. And quickly. If you believe you can't create a healthy lifestyle for yourself, then you're right. Before trying to attack your diet or your fitness, start by eliminating the negative belief holding you back.

Improve the thoughts you have about your journey and the words you use to describe it. Simple switches from "I have to" to "I get to" create an unstoppable change once you put it into practice. Learn to speak from gratitude and not from discontent.

Upgrade your standards

You will always get what you tolerate. Make sure you tolerate less and expect more of yourself. Upgrade to standards in line with your goals. If your goal is to lose 50 pounds and your standard of eating allows for unhealthy food choices, raise the bar. And I don't mean candy bar.

Upgrade your Circle of Success

Look at the people around you. You better believe you are the average of the five people with whom you spend the most time. Are you the outlier elevating the average? If so, you're in the wrong crew. Find people willing to help you grow. Break away from the ones holding you back. Upgrade to like-minded people who will not only show you the way, but will also walk the path with you.

Upgrade your love for the process

Stop fawning over fad diets and get-thin-quick schemes. Commit yourself to a process designed to change you from the inside. Fall in love with the work and understand the payoff isn't your achievements, it's the person you *become* in the process.

Upgrade your work ethic

Who are you when no one's looking? What you do behind closed doors will create amazing results when you step out into the public. Work your ass off, but do it for yourself. When you do it for yourself, you won't have to worry about who's watching while you work. You'll be watching, and you won't want to let yourself down.

Upgrade your nutrition

This book stands on the premise that your success in committing to a healthy lifestyle is 80% mindset and 20% mechanics. Your nutrition makes up a good portion of the mechanical 20% and should be addressed accordingly. Given the research outlined in this book about sugar addictions and how they can destroy your psyche and physiology, taking in quality nutrition is a MUST.

Upgrade your coaches and mentors

Find people who have done it before and can lead the way. In fitness, nutrition, life, and business, there is always room for growth and expansion. Leverage the experience of a coach or mentor to accelerate your progress while keeping you laser-focused on your goals. I happen to know a guy if you're looking for someone (www.JOINTHETH-RIVETRIBE.com).

UPGRADE YOUR LIFE!

You deserve an upgrade. You owe it to yourself. You're the only one who has a stake in your transformation.

It won't be a quick fix or a 30-second download. It's going to take time, effort, and consistency. I promise it will be worth it.

Testimonials from the Thrive Tribe

Meet Kelly H:

Two years ago, my friend SK started talking about this new program she had joined and her new trainer. Blah, blah, blah, we've heard it all before. How many trainers has she had now? How many diets? We've all watched her try time and again, and as usual, we wished her the best.

About six months into her new journey, I started to notice something different in her. She was sticking with it and really trying hard this time. She logged her food in her journal, thought about what she was eating, and was actually working out 5–6 days a week. I was proud of her, but also curious. After hearing so much about Jay and the "Thrive Tribe," I decided to dive in.

I showed up, all 220 out-of-shape pounds of me, workout gear on, water bottle and towel in hand, ready to meet the infamous Jay Nixon! I have to tell ya, it was fairly uneventful. He was a normal looking dude, no halo, no Dwayne Johnson muscles, no magic shoes to walk on water, just a guy. That first workout was horrible! I felt clumsy and out of shape and was highly embarrassed at my poor showing. I had to keep going; I promised six weeks of this nonsense.

Let's jump forward a year: a six-week promise turned into over a year, one workout a week turned into six workouts every week, and 220 pounds turned into 155 pounds! But, here's what really happened in the course of a year.

I fell into the lifestyle. I plan meals and stay within my calorie and carb goals every day. I enjoy getting up at 4:00 a.m. and working out every day. I am part of a tribe of support and purpose. I am on my way to becoming the best version of myself I can be.

Jay and the Tribe have helped me make a gigantic shift in mindset, attitude, purpose, and determination. The weekly calls keep us all on track and focused each week. The sharing of our struggles and victories with each other gives us purpose and drive. The community we have built allows us growth and commitment, not just to ourselves, but to others.

Jay's Journal

Today I will be my best and bring excellence to every situation that comes my way. Today, I will focus on upgrading myself—the way I speak, the way I think, and the way I behave. By consistently bettering myself in these areas, I will operate with a sense of purpose, which will allow me to be my best self.

Your Journal

_____

_____

_____

_____

_____

_____

Actions to Overcome the Overweight Mind

It's one thing to think about upgrading certain areas of your life, but nothing beats action. Below, you will be writing down three upgrades you need in your life. Don't take these lightly. Be mindful of the changes you want to make and be clear about why you need to change. Since we're nearing the end of the book, I'm giving you three **POWER Actions** to close this thing out strong. Don't quit on me now!

POWER Action 1: Fitness – Write down one upgrade you need to make in your fitness. Perhaps more exercise, keeping better track of your experiences, hiring a trainer to hold you accountable.

Power Action 2: Nutrition – Write down one upgrade you need to make for your nutrition. Do you need to rid your house of cookies and candy? Do you need to stop eating after a certain time? Should you upgrade your morning meal (get that protein shake in)? Choose wisely!

POWER Action 3: Relationships – Write down one relationship upgrade you need. How about better communication with your partner, calling your mom more often, mending fences with an old friend or family members. Make it count!

More Stories From Thrive Tribe Members Who Have Conquered the Overweight Mind

My journey with Jay Nixon began in July of 2015. I had noticed the progress of an acquaintance, Julie Kathawa, when our paths would cross at school drop-off in the mornings. I had asked her in January of 2015 what she was doing to look so fabulous. She invited me to come to Thrive and I was excited.

It wasn't until July 2015 that I walked through the doors of Thrive Fitness Studio, in Palm Desert, CA.

During my very first class with Jay, I knew I was in the right place. As I was trying not to run out of breath, I noticed he uses Doterra Essential oils and is diffusing them as we work out! Essential oils are a passion of mine and I use them daily. I had completed my first class and I was hooked. Jay uses a piece of equipment called the Power Plate. I had never heard of this before. He explained the benefits and uses of the Power Plates and how he uses them at Thrive. Everything was different in this studio. This was my beginning.

There are all different levels of fitness working together at the same time. As I attended each class, Jay performed his assessment and asked me, "What number on the scale would make you happy?" Well, I had hovered around

120-125 all my life. At my heaviest, without being pregnant, I weighed 150 pounds 20 years ago. At five feet tall, I never felt comfortable in my skin at that weight. I have had four children, six pregnancies and two C-sections, with one set of twins. My body has endured a lot. At 44 years old, I needed to get healthy to keep up with my children. I said 110 would make me happy. So, my journey began.

What I had noticed as I continue training with Jay and the Tribe was that this man does not allow negativity in his studio! He eliminates it and it doesn't exist at all. Never have I been to a gym where that was the case. I signed up for Jay's Come Alive and Thrive program, a six-week program designed to get me on the right track. The missing piece for me was accountability! We have partners as well as individual daily challenges at Thrive. The food menus are suggested and reviewed. We post on Facebook in our private group three things we are thankful for daily. As I continued on the program, I noticed the weight steadily decreasing. After about six months I was at 115. After one year, I hit my goal. I noticed I felt no "lighter" at 110 than I did at 126! How can that be? The scale said 110. What was going on?

So, I continued with six-week challenges and eating clean. My weight after about 15 months is 102! I have not weighed 102 since grade school. I feel strong and I know I am healthy. This July 2017 will be my two-year anniversary with the Tribe. My challenge now is to grow stronger mentally, write down my goals, and reach them. Jay has taught me to believe in myself. He gives us the tools to grow mentally and physically. We shed pounds, we laugh, and we cry tears of joy together at Thrive. We encourage one another daily. We bust through goals and create new ones.

As the Tribe has grown significantly in size over the last few years, so have the challenges he gives us. There is no such thing as a plateau at Thrive Fitness Studio.

I wanted to share my piece of the Thrive story. I am truly thankful I asked Julie what she was doing to look so good that morning at school drop-off. It truly changed my life. I am looking forward to what Thrive Fitness and Jay Nixon have in store for me as 2017 progresses and in the future. The decision I made that day to change for the better, to live better, and to do better was the beginning. I came alive the day I decided to come to Alive and Thrive with Jay Nixon. Forever grateful!

– Mary

**

Everybody has a story. Some want to share it and some want to keep it tucked away so no one can ever see or hear it. Well, I'm neither one of those. I want to SHOUT it from the rooftops so everyone can hear it and maybe be better because of it.

I was a 43-year-old working mother of three when I met Jay. I had never really cooked a day in my life and the running joke with my friends and family was the only reason I had a kitchen was because it came with the house. I had always—always—been overweight. Not obese, but always carrying 20–30 extra pounds. The one thing I never lacked though was self-confidence, which I needed every time I tried a new diet, and I tried them ALL: Jenny Craig, Weight Watchers, Lindora, the Hollywood Diet, the cookie diet (trust me, not as good as it sounds), Nutrisystem, and even the "just not eating" diet.

I tried and failed every single time over a 24-year span. It wasn't until I met Jay and went through his six-week program I finally "got it." He taught me I needed to change the way I viewed food and how food was actually affecting me and my body. Honestly, I thought a bagel and cream cheese was a healthy choice, that I could eat as much fruit as I wanted. I mean it's fruit, right? Jay taught me what different foods actually do to you, how the body processes them, and how they are good or bad for you when trying to lose weight. It might seem simple to you, but for me it was groundbreaking information no one had ever taught me in any of my weight-loss endeavors. It felt amazing to GET IT!

I was just two and a half weeks into this process and I went out to dinner and a concert to celebrate my sister's birthday (she's in this book and she is AWESOME). I chose healthy food, chose not to drink, and felt completely satisfied. As I sat in my seat waiting for the concert to start, I got so giddy (it's really how I felt), I said to myself "I'm finally going to be thin." Little did I know I was going to be more than just thin. I was going to be the best version of myself. I did know in that short period of time, however, this was the real deal. This guy was the real deal. This was going to be life changing. I was so engaged and so willing to do whatever it took to get healthy.

So, why did this work when other programs failed? Jay taught me to change my mindset, not only with food but in all aspects of my life also. Now, I hold myself to a higher standard, not only with my diet and exercise but also with my relationships, with my business practices, and even in my parenting. He has taught me to be my best self. I strive for every day to be better than the last. It's an exciting process and I love everything about it. Now I use my kitchen to make healthy meals to nourish my family as I try and mold three children to be their best selves.

— Julie

**

I am in the early stages of my personal journey with Jay and the Tribe (less than six months), so I'd like to focus on the profound mental impact Jay has had on my life already. I was on Facebook one night and started reading testimonies from friends in the community about Jay's program, and how he has positively changed their lives.

I immediately knew I needed to see what this was all about because I was yearning for a place that could help me change and become healthier as soon as possible.

After having a discussion about the program with my husband, I walked into Thrive to register and become a member. The day I walked into the studio, I had already hit rock bottom. I was extremely depressed, anxious, and desperate to get myself out of the hole I had been in for nearly three years. I was very overweight, but even worse, I was extremely afraid about the direction my health was headed. I wasn't taking care of myself, and sadly, I didn't LOVE myself.

Taking the first step was difficult, especially standing on the scale and having reality sink in. Fortunately, Jay's approach as a trainer is very nonjudgmental, and he is the most motivating person I have ever met in my life. It was very humbling in the beginning, always being the last one to finish, and constantly working through the sore muscles. But, before I knew it, there would be another new Tribe member joining, and my role would be changing, as I would be the one cheering on somebody else new and in a vulnerable position.

Jay has created a tribe where members support one another and build each other up. His program will not tolerate any criticism or negativity. I have changed as a person, because Jay teaches us to start each day with gratitude and positivity. He has made me realize when I wake up feeling thankful, the rest of my day is bound to be great!

I have tried so many different approaches out there: Jenny Craig, Weight Watchers, Shakeology, CrossFit, and going to the gym by myself. Nothing comes remotely close to Jay's Thrive Tribe. I have such a sense of relief and feel so fortunate that I have found this tribe. It is so comforting to me, knowing I can have this support system for life.

As a registered nurse working in the healthcare industry, it takes a lot for me to trust and to be convinced when I'm starting something new in life. Jay is very knowledgeable about nutrition, fitness, and the physiology of the human body and mind. I am most impressed Jay is constantly furthering his own knowledge as well by following great mentors and attending seminars.

Jay's weekly phone calls have been very therapeutic for me. He has such a way of delivering very powerful messages about bettering my life. Since I have joined Thrive, I have learned not to let stress take over my life. I used to get derailed and turn to food for comfort. Jay has helped me identify that food is only about providing fuel and nutrition, not comfort. I have also learned a lot more about my addiction to sugar—how sugar is basically poison. I have realized I no longer want to be causing chronic inflammation throughout my body, whether it's from sugar or dairy consumption. Being a part of Thrive has not only been about exercise or losing weight, but it has also furthered my knowledge about living my best life. I am eager to start spreading this important knowledge so it will have a positive impact on the rest of my family, and, most importantly, on my children.

I have lost a solid 17 pounds forever, and I can't wait to reach 20 pounds. After that, I will continue setting more weight-loss goals. Jay has emphasized this journey is a process and to be patient. After all, I didn't gain all of this weight in just six months! This program is not about finding a quick fix. It is about embarking on an amazing, fulfilling journey for life.

Thankfully, I am no longer alone in my battle for health and fitness because I have a wonderful, amazing tribe where everyone shares the same goals and mutual respect for one another. I no longer feel depressed or anxious. In less than six months, I am without any medications! I can even say that I LOVE myself again!

Jay makes himself available for moral support to any Tribe member when needed. Jay has helped me realize I am important, and that I deserve to take care of myself instead of just taking care of others all of the time. I am so eager and optimistic to see what my future hold. Now I know the sky's the limit, simply because I have Jay and the Thrive Tribe in my life.

– Maggie S.

**

Growing up in a small town in Montana, my earliest memories are of always being a "fat kid." At age eight, I remember being in a room and playing with toys while a person I did not know asked me questions. Later in my life, I asked my parents about the visit and my mother let me know they had taken me to a weight-loss doctor. I know my weight has always been directly a result of inappropriate eating patterns over many decades. When I was in elementary school, my grandpa would pick me up every day for lunch. He would take me to my house and I would eat lunch. We would then go to his house and I would eat a second meal upon my grandma's insistence. My grandma would not let me leave the table until my plate was clear. Of course, she did not know how to cook healthy meals. Everything *was fried and in huge portions. I also remember my grandmother made most of my clothes.*

When I got into middle school, it became obvious I was overweight. I was teased by many of my classmates. I never felt like I fit in. I would try to lose weight, but the only way I knew how to do it was not to eat. Of course that never worked. Another major issue I had most of my life was the clothes I had to buy. I was never able to find stylish clothes in my size. It was embarrassing having to go to the big sizes to try to find items that would fit. Because of my weight, I was always chosen last for games in PE, which was extremely embarrassing and made me feel worthless. Every year I would intentionally make sure I had some knee or ankle injury so I didn't have to participate in PE class. It was a vicious cycle lasting throughout my high school years. During high school, I tried multiple times to "diet"/ starve myself so I would fit in with everyone else. Nothing changed during my high school years. I really didn't fit in and I could never get my weight under control.

In my first semester of college, I was so homesick I couldn't eat. This was the first time I was able to lose any amount of weight. I then met my soon-to-be-husband and quickly realized he was the first person to love me for me with no mention of my weight. I kept my weight off for about two years by eating relatively healthily, but not exercising. Exercising was never in my vocabulary, and I really didn't know what to do.

My husband was a college athlete and always wanted me to spend time with him working out, but I refused because of the negative experiences I'd had most of my life. Slowly, after having two children, going to college, and beginning work, my weight returned.

After the birth of my second son, I had gained over 70 pounds. I tried every diet possible to get the weight off, but it was just a vicious cycle. I would lose weight, then put back on more weight.

By the time my older son was a senior in high school, I weighed more than I ever had and I felt totally helpless. I decided to look into weight-loss surgery because I didn't know what else to do. I also felt it was time to focus on me instead of everyone else. I thought weight-loss surgery would be the easy way out. I finally had the surgery. I did lose over 100 pounds, but I also had several complications. Within a six-month time frame, I had to have three more surgeries. At the beginning this was a great "tool," but there was no permanent fix. It is not easy to keep the weight off, and it still is a daily struggle.

Right after the surgery (for the first time in my life), I joined a gym and got a personal trainer. My trainer helped me realize my health was of utmost importance. We worked together for two years and I was the strongest and the thinnest that I had ever been, and I finally felt good about myself. My trainer left and went back to school, and I lost my direction. I started to gain weight again because I had no accountability. I was not strong enough by myself to say no to unhealthy food choices.

Both of my children were out of the house and I felt it was time to focus on me. I reached out to Jay Nixon because I had been watching several people and their transformations. From day one it was like something I had never experienced before. Everyone at his studio is so encouraging and willing to help in any way possible. I feel like I belong to a family. Jay is so motivating and makes me feel like I can do anything. In the little amount of time I have been a part of the "Tribe," I feel like a totally different person. I am beginning to realize who I really am and what I am capable of doing. I love the daily expectations. I am inspired daily to be the best person I can be both mentally and physically, continually encouraged by all of the "Thrive Tribe" members. Jay Nixon's ability to communicate in a no-nonsense way while being inspiring, has changed my life.

– Mardi H.

**

I was lucky enough to be born into a family with three other siblings. I have a sister who is eight years older than I am, a brother four years older, and my twin brother. When I was about eight years old, my parents asked us what we wanted to be when we grew up. My brothers wanted to be a professional football player and a doctor and my sister wanted to be Miss America. She was sixteen at the time and I idolized her. She was tall, slim, and loved to model. When it was my turn to answer, the first thing that popped into my head was, "I want to be skinny when I grow up." But I never told them that. I gave the obligatory answer: "a lawyer." That's my earliest memory of being self-conscious about my body image. I wasn't even overweight, but compared to my siblings, I was the "chubby" one.

I think I was about eleven when my mom asked me if I wanted to go on a diet with her for the first time. She liked to try every diet under the sun. It was the beginning of a new year and she had her resolutions. I remember feeling very sad after she asked me, and I had a ton of questions running through my head. "Does she think I'm fat?" "Is she embarrassed by me?"

She obviously didn't ask my sister who was thin. I reluctantly agreed, and we tried the latest fad diet for about a month and then quit and so my dieting odyssey began, a vicious cycle of fad diets. I would lose some weight, then gain it back after...and so on. Exercise was never a component.

This had pretty much been my life for the last 20 years until I woke up one morning less than 2 years ago realizing I was the heaviest I had ever been and I needed to do something about it. I was 160 lbs and was barely fitting into a size 12. My youngest child was almost five and I was out of excuses. A friend of mine introduced me to Jay and my life has changed forever.

My initial goal after meeting with Jay for the first time was solely weight loss. Before I met Jay, I was exercising maybe once a week (that's being generous). So, I joined my first six-week program and I began going to his 8:30 a.m. class on Tuesdays and Thursdays. As hard as it was, the days I wasn't exercising at Thrive, I missed it. So I changed my days to Mondays, Wednesdays, and Fridays. I even started to add Saturdays here and there. One day my friend said, "You should come to the 5:15 a.m. class!" I laughed and said, "You will never catch me at a 5:15 a.m. class...that's just way too early to work out!"

Then, one morning Jay said something I will never forget: "You need to learn to be comfortable with the uncomfortable!" From that one conversation, I decided I was going to try a 5:15 a.m. class. I showed up on Monday at 5:15 a.m....and then again on Tuesday... and then again on Wednesday...throughout the rest of the week! I couldn't believe it! I was so uncomfortable showing up so early, but I did and I loved it. From then on, I was hooked! For the last year and a half I have worked out with Jay and the Tribe six days a week. I work out Monday through Friday at 5:15 a.m. and Saturday at 6:15 a.m.! As long as I am in town, I show up.

I am now 130 lbs and fit loosely into a size four! I have new goals in hand. When I think back to my first initial meeting with Jay, I giggle a little. My goal was solely weight loss... but Jay and his Thrive Tribe are SOOOO much more than that. I have learned how to fall in love with exercising. I learned why none of those diets I did throughout my life worked...because it isn't about "dieting," it's about a lifestyle change. I have been doing back-to-back six-week challenges since I met Jay. I have learned that even though I exercise six days a week, I can't out-exercise bad eating. I have gained the tools and the knowledge to be the best possible version of myself.

But, the most important thing of all, I have learned to love myself… and the best feeling in the world is when I get home from my early morning workouts and my kids tell me they are so proud to have the strongest mommy in the world.

– Rachel B

**

I met Jay 15 days after my 47th birthday. My sister, Julie, was halfway through her six-week challenge with Jay. She would not stop bugging me about him. She would call me almost every day and tell me I needed to do this program with her in February. Seriously, she would not let up. At the time my petite, 5'1" frame was carrying around 262 pounds, and I had been overweight or obese for the last 35 years.

She kept telling me this program was different. Did I believe her for a second? Nope, I did not, but I did finally sign up just to get her the heck off my back. What did I have to lose, right? That's the best part of my story…I lost weight, but I gained so much more. I gained the knowledge, tools, and mindset that will keep me from ever being overweight again. Ever! And I learned I deserve to be my best self every day!

You're probably thinking: "Well I can't do that. It's too hard for me. I can't walk because my knees hurt or I can't do a jumping jack. I'll never be able to work out for half an hour at a time." That was me.

I know you. I was you.

I have tried every diet out there. When I was 12, I did the Atkins diet with my dad. When I was 13, I went to the diet center with my mom. When I was 16, I tried a diet that included B-12 shots. There was even a diet where we wore a belt with a little bump on it that pushed into our stomachs to keep us from being hungry, kind of like an exterior gastric bypass.

When I graduated from high school and went off on my own, I did Jenny Craig. I did SlimFast. I did Weight Watchers. I even did a medically-supervised, liquid fasting diet through the local hospital. Every diet you can imagine I've been on, and I was successful. I lost weight on every diet but I never got to my goal weight and eventually gained every pound back plus more. I've yo-yo dieted for the last 35 years.

I know you. I was you.

This is not a diet. This is a lifestyle change. This is a mindset change. This is something that will make you the happiest and healthiest you have ever been. I'm a type-1 diabetic. I've been diabetic since I was 19. Pretty late for juvenile diabetes, but it happened to me. Since that time, I have never been less than 160 pounds. From the time I was 19, I worried about the complications I would face because of my diabetes: kidney failure and dialysis; loss of toes, feet, and legs; glaucoma; heart disease; neuropathy.

About a month before I heard about Jay, I was sitting on the floor in front of my open refrigerator drinking orange juice and trying to raise my blood sugar enough to stop the convulsions. When the episode was over I was lying in a pool of orange juice, sweating and crying and praying to God to help me. I asked for help with getting control over my constant battles with food and the high and low blood sugars that went along with them.

I knew they would be the death of me. I spent almost 30 years worrying about the battles but I never did anything to prevent them.

Until now! With Jay's instruction I have finally figured out what food is for. It is fuel for our body. It keeps our bodies moving and active. It's for making sure we are healthy. It's for stopping the hunger pains. That's it. Food is meant to be consumed to nourish our bodies and to keep us healthy and strong. I did not know it at the time, but God answered my prayer in the form of Jay Nixon and this program.

When I first met Jay I remember thinking, "This guy is nuts. He tells me I won't miss bread or Girl Scout cookies." All I could think was he's crazy. The thing is, he's not. Everything he said to me during our first meeting happened. Everything. I haven't eaten McDonald's food in 23 months and I don't miss it at all. It is pretty easy to bypass all the processed sweets and treats because I know now they are unnecessary and unhealthy. Homemade treats are harder to pass up because they are not processed, but through this program I have raised my standards and do not indulge every time I'm offered a treat.

I have been working with Jay for almost two years now. I'm going to tell you a hard truth—the beginning was hard. Really hard. I craved everything from bread to candy to chips. It was hard to eat vegetables. I only ate green beans and asparagus. I missed my diet sodas, too. Then, something clicked. My body started craving veggies. I started making Brussels sprouts, spaghetti squash, zucchini, and cauliflower. They tasted delicious. I crave them now like I used to crave sugar treats. When I had a reward meal and drank a Diet Pepsi my taste buds said, "Blah, this is terrible." I haven't had one since. Your body starts to recognize the difference between real, clean food and nasty, processed food filled with chemicals.

The best parts of this program are the mental cleansing and the mindset shift that occur. It's been a struggle to get my mind to believe I am capable and that I deserve to be a beautiful, healthy woman. I am smart enough, strong enough, and deserving enough to get whatever I desire in life. Because of Jay and this program, I have lost 104 pounds and have gained my life back. I was on my way to killing myself using food as my weapon of choice. As a type-1 diabetic, I knew I was fast approaching the point where my body was going to start rebelling from the years of abuse I had been forcing on it.

Jay gives you all the tools you will need to succeed at this lifestyle change. If I can do this and I can lose more than 100 pounds, anyone can do this. Do not let another minute of your life go by without taking the plunge. It was, hands-down, the absolute best decision I've ever made. I thank my sister constantly for giving me the push to get me to sign up, and I thank God every day for sending me Jay Nixon.

I know you. I was you.

This is not a diet. It's a lifestyle change. If you take the leap and jump into this with both feet, you will be successful. You will become happier and healthier every day.

– Sylvia

**

On May 15, 2013, the first version of my story began. I walked into labor and delivery as a strong, fierce, glowing, bubbly, and very pregnant first-time mom. I was going in for a scheduled induction and was about to meet our son. After 26 hours of labor and an emergency C-section, our precious Owen Thomas took his first breath with the assistance of many machines. He was taken from my belly and immediately rushed next door to CHLA to undergo the first of several, open-heart surgeries. I was determined to get released to join my new family, and in 30 hours I walked out of the hospital with hope.

What met me was a world I could have never imagined. Our son was one day old, post-op, and swollen, with tubes and lines everywhere. His chest and small body were covered and his eyes were shielded from the bright lights. I remember seeing him for the first time and thinking, "How could this tiny human be my perfect baby?" When I saw his fight, I instantly fell deeply and madly in love with him. We made sure each one of Owen's 112 days on this earth were filled with nothing but color, joy and love despite the medication, procedures, surgeries, and difficulties he would experience daily—treatments to which we had to give consent..

Devastatingly, on September 4, 2013, Owen no longer needed to fight and he was wholly healed when he left this world for the next, awaiting our reunion. When he left, he took my joy, fight, and glow with him. Two months later, the first of two rainbows (Owen's gifts) came to us when I found myself pregnant with our second son. The pregnancy was full of anxiety and constant fear. But, when Brody came into this world, I was determined to show him the same love and joy we showed our first. I pressured myself to push away and hide the sadness and focus only on our healthy boy. While I held our son close to my chest, I feared he would be taken away. In fact, this fear poured out to all of my relationships. I watched as friends disappeared and a gap started to form with my husband. We were existing in sleepless nights and days filled with questions as second-time, first-time parents.

Eighteen months later we welcomed our third son, our second Band-Aid. He came into a world of chaos and uncertainty. I was beyond grateful for *my gifts, had an incredibly loving, attentive, and supportive husband, and was madly in love with our sons, but there was still a hole that could not be filled and a light that was so dim, I was sure it had just gone out. When my third son was five months old, I was getting out of the shower and paused in front of the mirror. I did not recognize the woman staring back at me. She was exhausted, pale, sad, lost, angry and, most of all, desperate to feel alive again.*

I reached out to a friend and she told me about the Thrive Tribe. I was scared to death to make the first call but knew I needed to make a change. The next day, I walked in the door of the studio with my son in his infant car seat and said, "HELP!" The first day I was filled with fear and the workout was excruciating. The second workout, even worse! But, as the days went on, the new version of my story began. I felt exhaustion steadily replaced by pride in myself. I felt fear being replaced by strength. I let moments of PTSD become moments of inspiration.

I meet daily with a group of positive people whose light has relit my flame and made me unstoppable. I let go of anger and replaced it with love and kindness. I took the hard shell that had formed and became vulnerable as I softened myself to those who earned my trust and worked to protect me. Six months into my new story, I'm 33 pounds lighter, I'm free of an immeasurable amount of emotional baggage, stand taller, love more fiercely, welcome spontaneity, laugh genuinely, and, most of all, love the strong, brave, powerful, toned, and beautiful woman I see in the mirror looking back at me. I'm eternally grateful for Jay Nixon and the Tribe.

– Alissa V.

**

I can remember sitting in my car and crying in front of the new juice bar after hanging up from my first phone call with Jay. I thought to myself, "Finally. I think this guy might actually be able to help me, but I am terrified."

I was in a very miserable state! I was very overweight. Pants and underwear were cutting off my circulation, and I had to unbutton my pants when I sat in the car and at my desk at work. I felt like my skin was too tight and my clothes were even tighter. I felt terrible, depressed, and unhealthy. I was in my office alone one day, eating a spinach salad and I choked. I choked on spinach! I couldn't breathe, I was alone and so scared. After the first episode, I started choking all of the time. I couldn't eat anything without throwing it up, I couldn't even hold water down. I couldn't eat dinner and lie down. The food would come right back up. I ended up going to the doctor. My blood pressure was 180/105. After a series of tests, I was diagnosed with severe reflux and high blood pressure. I received prescription after prescription. I could not go one day without my medication or I would choke or throw up my food/water. This absolutely scared the shit out of me. It made me feel like I was going to die and leave my children without a mother. The absolute worst feeling ever.

Thank goodness I was fortunate enough to meet Jay. His guidance and support have helped me become prescription free! I wish the doctors were able to write a prescription for all patients to enroll in Jay's program. It is much more beneficial than anything else doctors can write on a pad. I feel so much better. Now instead of ordering that fruit bowl with granola I "thought" was good for me, I know what I can order and what will truly benefit by body. I would write more, but my story isn't over. I still have a lot to learn and a lot to accomplish for myself.

– Cindy R.

Support My Mission To Help A Million People

By reading The Overweight Mind, you are now a member of the Tribe. I believe one of our greatest gifts is the ability to help others on their journey. It only takes one person's story to change the lives of hundreds or even thousands, and your story could do just that.

If this book resonated with you and helped you on your journey, please go to Amazon and leave a detailed review. My mission is to help people live the life they deserve to live, and now you can be a part of that process by sharing your story for others to read.

Simply scroll down to the book page on Amazon and click "Write A Customer Review" - know that each review greatly appreciated and that I am grateful beyond words for your help in spreading my mission and message.

If you'd like to stay in touch with the Tribe and get additional resource to help you live your best life make sure you checkout:

The Overweight Mind
www.TheOverweightMind.com

About the Author

Jay Nixon is a speaker, author, mentor, and coach whose mission is to help each and every person achieve their "absolute best self." He is the owner of the Thrive Fitness Studio in Palm Desert, California, and the grateful leader of the Thrive Tribe, a collection of Jay's current and former clients who work together to improve their health, their fitness, and their lives.

For over two decades, Jay has helped thousands of people achieve total body transformation through a cohesive combination of fitness, nutrition, and personal development coaching. Jay believes, "If you give people the right tools, education, and support, they can far surpass what they once thought was their maximum potential." He's known for his innate ability to get inside someone's head, helping him/her achieve life-changing results.

Recognized as a lululemon Ambassador and dubbed by CBS News as, "One of the best fitness and nutrition experts in the business," Jay has been featured on ABC and FOX, and in *Triathlete* magazine. When he's not working with clients one-on-one, you'll find him consulting for Fortune 1000 companies in the nutrition and fitness industry. Learn more at www.NixonElite.com.

References for The Overweight Mind

» www.muscleprodigy.com/michael-phelps-workout-and-diet/

» www.psychologytoday.com/blog/the-science-willpower/200912/
sugar-addiction-in-your-body-not-just-your-mind

» www.espn.com/blog/denver-broncos/post/_/id/19274/
transcript-of-peyton-mannings-retirement-speech

» www.youtube.com/watch?v=ub_a2t0ZfTs

» www.independent.co.uk/news/science/sugar-has-similar-effect-on-brain-as-cocaine-a6980336.html

» www.slate.com/articles/health_and_science/science/2013/07/what_is_dopamine_love_lust_sex_addiction_gambling_motivation_reward.html

» www.ncbi.nlm.nih.gov/pmc/articles/PMC2769828/

» www.webmd.com/diabetes/type-2-diabetes-guide/type-2-diabetes#1

» professional.diabetes.org/sites/professional.diabetes.org/files/media/fast_facts_12-2015a.pdf

» www.espn.com/mma/fighter/history/_/id/2563796/ronda-rousey

» www.espn.com/espnw/sports/article/18379890/
in-quest-revenge-pride-ronda-rousey-lost-own-way

» www.niddk.nih.gov/health-information/health-statistics/Pages/over-weight-obesity-statistics.aspx

» www.nytimes.com/2016/05/02/health/biggest-loser-weight-loss.html?_r=0

» www.eonline.com/news/813640/the-biggest-loser-winner-ali-vincent-speaks-out-after-regaining-weight-i-don-t-know-if-i-ever-believed-in-myself

» jamanetwork.com/journals/jamasurgery/fullarticle/2422341

» www.refme.com/us/citation-generator/apa/

» www.ucl.ac.uk/news/news-articles/0908/09080401

»   www.habitsforwellbeing.com/6-core-human-needs-by-anthony-robbins/

»   www.history.com/this-day-in-history/
     roger-bannister-breaks-four-minutes-mile

»   www.nfl.com/player/demarcomurray/2495207/careerstats

»   www.trackandfieldnews.com/index.php/
     category-stats/1932-splits-in-world-record-miles

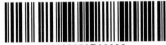

Made in the USA
San Bernardino, CA
28 August 2017